Only the Essentials

A Concise Aromatherapy Reference Guide

Michele A. Williams, R.Ph.

Aroma Rx®, Inc.
Los Alamos, California

Only the Essentials:
A Concise Aromatherapy Reference Guide
By Michele A. Williams

Printed in the United States of America
First Printing 2004

ISBN: 0-974923-80-X
Library of Congress Control Number: 2004094429

Published by:
Aroma Rx®, Inc.
PO Box 331
Los Alamos, CA 93440 U.S.A.
(805) 344-1314
Fax: (805) 344-1334
Email: info@aromarx.com
Web: www.aromarx.com

Book Layout and Cover Design by Odyssey Marketing Group
Photography by David Lloyd
Printed and Bound by Kudzu Graphics
Proofreading by Paula Engel
Publishing Consulting by Gordon Burgett
Special Thanks to North Fulton Apothecary Compounding Pharmacy

Disclaimer

Healing and medicine are two distinct fields, and the law requires this disclaimer. This booklet is an educational reference work based on collation of current literature and the author's personal experience. Any slights of people or organizations are unintentional. The content of this book is not intended as medical advice, or to diagnose, prescribe, or treat any illness, disease, or condition of the body or mind. The information therein is in no way to be considered as a substitute for consultation with a licensed medical practitioner.

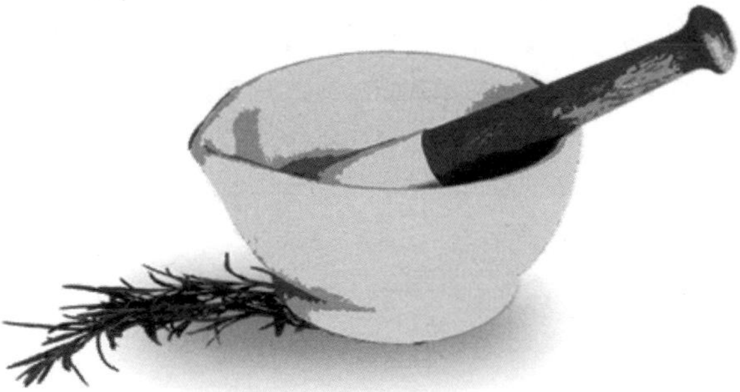

Karen –
Blessings for perfect
health, prosperity & joy!
Michelle Williams

I am grateful to Spirit
that abundantly provides me inspiration and wisdom.

I thank Mom, Dad, and Aileen
for their constant and perfect love and support.

I appreciate my health and vitality
and it is my joy to share
these gifts via the content of this book.

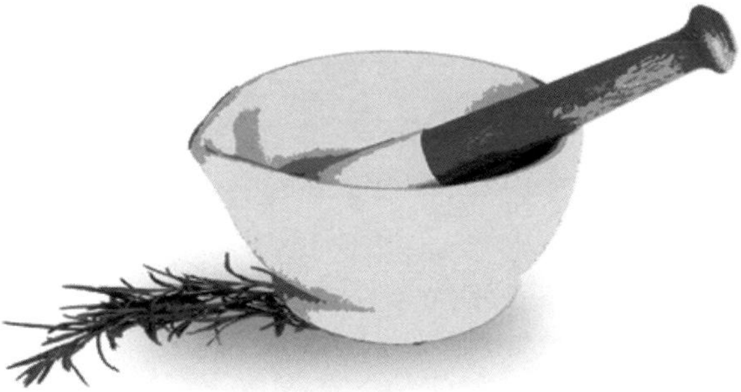

About the Author

With over nineteen years of clinical pharmacy experience, Michele Williams is one of a few pharmacists that specialize in aromatherapy and natural medicine.

Just two years after graduating pharmacy school and practicing pharmacy, Michele began to ask, "Why aren't people getting healthy using medications?" and "Do I have an unrealistic expectation of healthcare or about health in general?"

Michele was in the perfect place to discover these answers, being stationed in the United States Air Force at RAF Lakenheath, United Kingdom. She watched as some of her friends waited weeks to be seen by a physician through the Public Health System, while other friends used self-help treatments, such as herbs, homeopathy, Bach flower remedies, massage, etc. Michele noticed that these non-pharmaceutical approaches worked to help her friends get well more quickly and/or maintain their health.

Her training paradigm and skepticism had not prepared her to accept that such things as herbs (of all things!) or zinc lozenges or homeopathic remedies could eliminate colds and other ailments. What, no antibiotics? That was not the American approach! Funny thing though: people using these remedies got through their illnesses and did so quickly. What was going on?

Suspecting that there had to be something more than the placebo effect, Michele began her own journey of learning. Realizing that many pharmaceuticals are derived from plants, Michele surmised that there might be something to all this "herbs and stuff."

In 1992, Michele was introduced to essential oils through a reflexology practitioner who had been practicing aromatherapy for nearly fifteen years at that point. Michele was amazed at the subtle affects of these oils, their powerful healing actions, and the effects they produced on a person's mood and emotions. Michele learned about the therapeutic value of the oils and has been promoting their value ever since. She has come to appreciate holistic principles and the healing power of nature.

Michele continues to examine other natural medicine modalities such as chiropractic, massage, reflexology, Reiki, acupuncture, mind-body energy medicine, etc. Like many licensed practitioners that received allopathic training, Michele evaluates grandiose medical claims skeptically, but after fifteen years of continuous study of natural medicine and the holistic healing approach, she is firmly convinced that there are many valid ways of healing.

This is Michele's mission: to empower consumers to be their own best health advocates. She is passionate about bridging the gap between current western medicine and natural medicine. She strongly believes in a totally integrated approach to holistic health care, incorporating natural medicine (i.e., aromatherapy, herbs, vitamins, and nutraceuticals), nutrition, exercise, mind-body energy, spirituality, and, if necessary, pharmaceuticals, to mobilize the greatest potential for healing.

Michele is President and CEO of Aroma Rx®, Inc., and provides educational seminars and presentations on aromatherapy, holistic healing, and integrative medicine.

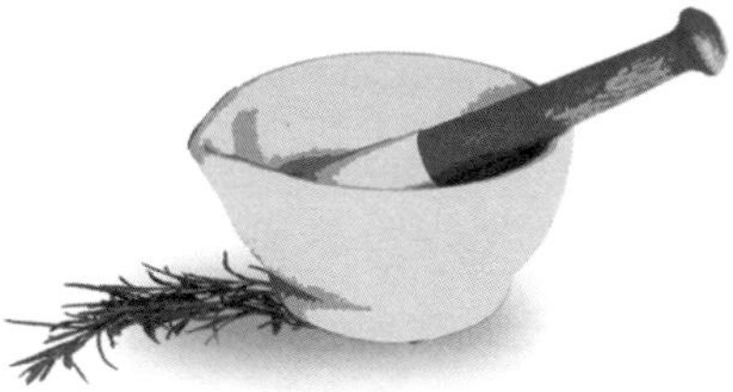

Contents

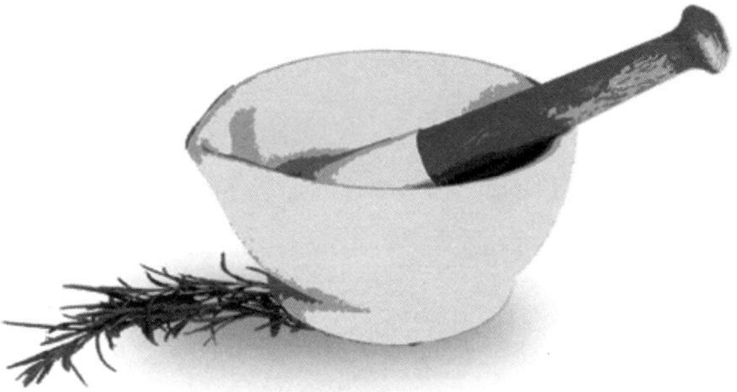

Preface

When I'm exposed to new ideas, I like to learn more about them, so I read. I believe information is best presented in a manner that's clean, concise, and accurate. The reader should be able to find the information easily and be able to understand it. My book and the title I chose for it, *Only the Essentials* is intended to accomplish just that. In addition, I want the experience of reading my book to be exciting, dynamic, and uplifting, as are the essential oils themselves.

After four years of focusing our wholesale business on integrative medicine clinics and natural medicine practitioners, Aroma Rx®, Inc. opened The Aroma Shoppe in Los Alamos, California, in September 2003. Our greatest demand from our customers continues to be for accurate, useful, and helpful information. *Only the Essentials: A Concise Aromatherapy Reference Guide* is an excellent guide for readers to intelligently incorporate scent into daily living. This book is invaluable to practicing massage therapists and aromatherapy practitioners needing a quick reference to essential oils and their indications. Lastly, this book serves as an indispensable learning and development tool to teach basic essential oil information to new employees responsible for sales of essential oils.

Although this book is not meant to be an all-inclusive education in aromatherapy, I have provided an extensive list of references for future reading. There are many knowledgeable authors and valuable books available on different aspects of aromatherapy, as well as various educational tools that provide in-depth study. I acknowledge and thank all of these wonderful people and resources who have been instrumental in bringing aromatherapy to its current thriving status today.

Aromatherapy is an ancient practice with a great deal of modern consumer interest, but practical questions still remain. To fill that need, this concise but comprehensive guide presents the basic principles of aromatherapy and provides the essential information you need to be able to incorporate those principles into your daily life safely, effectively, and enjoyably.

The heart of this book is a comprehensive list of 145 essential oils and 40 carrier oils which includes:

- Common and botanical name
- Scent, blending characteristics, and note type (for perfumery)
- Traditional and/or documented uses
- Applications
- Country of origin
- Distillation method
- Part of the plant used
- Precautions

There are also several convenient cross-reference charts and guides including a skin care oil guide and a glossary of terms.

It's not important which mechanism you choose to enter into the world of aromatherapy and healing. What matters is that you have taken the first step to be your own advocate in your health, vitality, well-being, and happiness.

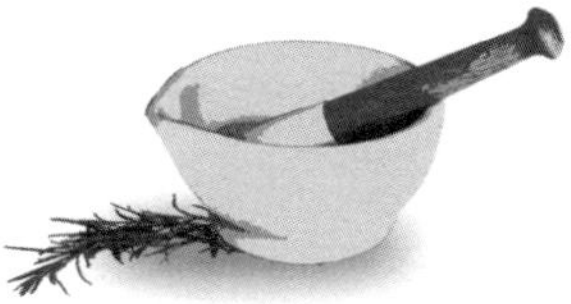

What is Aromatherapy?

As more people take responsibility for their healthcare, there is a growing impulse to utilize natural products for therapeutic and cosmetic benefits. Aromatherapy is a popular choice because of our receptivity to scent and its "feel good" advantages. "Aroma" products can be found in candles, shampoos, air fresheners, body soap, bath oils, cosmetics, and perfumes. To date, aromatherapy is the fastest growing healing art in this country.

Aromatherapy is the healing art and science that uses essential oils in a positive way to promote or maintain good health and to calm, balance, and rejuvenate the body, mind, and spirit. Essential oils are highly concentrated, volatile, natural substances extracted from specialized plant cells: the flower, leaf, blossom, petal, resin, tree, bark, root, twig, seed, berry, rind, and rhizome. They are considered "gems of nature," the "quintessential" life force, and the condensation of a plant's vital "essence"—the soul of the plant—in which is stored vital solar energy. This essential oil is what gives the plant its fragrance.

The highly concentrated essential oil holds most of the plant's valuable therapeutic properties. This essence is produced by special cells within the plant and contains vitamins and phytohormones that are sensitive to heat and light and are soluble in oil. Their tiny molecular structure penetrates in two ways: into the skin to the internal organs and through the olfactory nerves in the nose to the brain. They perform their effect both topically and internally.

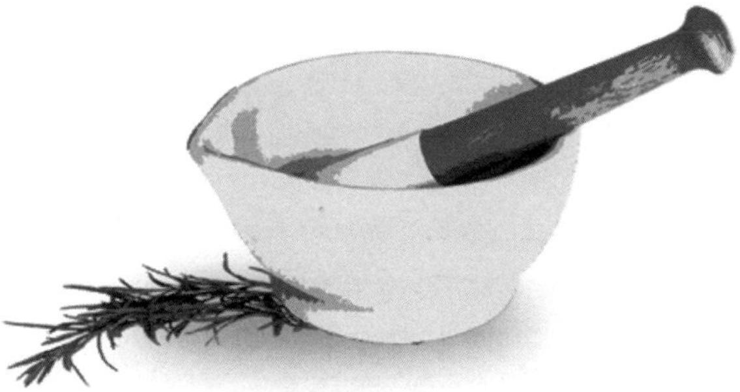

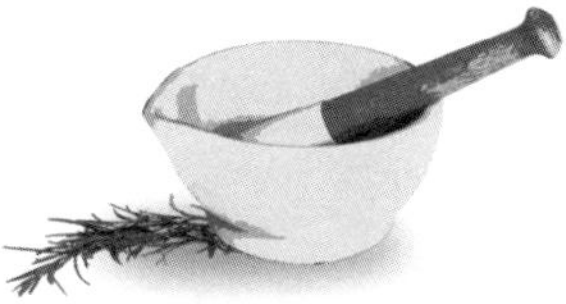

History of Modern Aromatherapy

In 500 BC, Hippocrates stated, "The way to health is to have an aromatic bath and scented massage every day." However, aromatherapy has even earlier origins. The oldest surviving Chinese pharmacopoeia, the Pen Ts'ao (*Divine Husbandman's Materia Medica*), attributed to Emperor Shen Nung, was composed around 2700 BC and contains information of over 300 aromatic herbs. Records indicate that the Indian practice of Ayurveda has used aromatic plants for over 3000 years. An Egyptian papyrus dated around 1550 BC details the use of aromatic plants as remedies. Additionally, there are over 180 references to oils in the Bible. One of the earliest ways of using aromatic extracts as offerings to their gods was as incense offered to gods. Egyptians also used fragrant oils for healing, embalming, purifying, and massage after bathing.

The Greeks continued the medicinal and cosmetic use of aromatic plant oils. The *De Materia Medica*, written by Pedacius Dioscorides, a Greek physician, was universally used in the Greek, Roman, and Arab worlds from the second century AD until modern times.

Imperial Rome became known as the "bathing capital of the world" through the proliferation of perfumes and oils carried by their extensive trade routes from Arabia and the Far East. Crusaders encountered these exotic oils in the Middle East and reintroduced them into Europe.

Avicenna, an Arab physician who lived from 980 to 1037 AD, is first credited with utilizing a process resembling modern methods of distillation to produce lighter perfumes that were not heavily based in oil.

During the Middle Ages, the antiseptic and bactericidal properties of plants were recognized and used extensively. The positive effects on the immune system appeared to combat the European Plague for some people.

With the accumulation of the antiseptic discoveries and the use of distillation in the 15th century, more aromatic plants were distilled to create essential oils. Books on herbs and their properties also began appearing. Paracelcus, an alchemist and medical doctor, is credited with coining the term "essence" as he focused upon using plants as medicines.

Oils could be purchased at "apothecaries" during the 16th century, and perfumery was clearly establishing a niche as its own art form. Through the 19th century, perfumery remained a prosperous industry. This was an important time scientifically as the major constituents of essential oils were isolated and identified.

Then in the 20th century, European scientists began researching the antibacterial effects of essential oils. Essential oils were used on the wounds of those who suffered in the terrible trench warfare of 1914-1918. In 1928, while researching the cosmetic applications of essential oils, the French cosmetic scientist Rene-Maurice Gattefosse wrote the first research paper in which the word "aromatherapie" was used. After he severely burned his hand in his laboratory, he plunged it in pure lavender oil. The oil at once eased his pain and the wound healed quickly, without infection or scarring. After this incident, Gattefosse turned his attention to the use of oils in dermatology and researched their potential medicinal uses as antiseptics and analgesics. He later set up a business producing oils for use in cosmetics.

Soon thereafter, Frenchman Albert Couvreur, published a book which discussed the medicinal application of essential oils. Simultaneously, other research began appearing independently from around the world. In Australia, the antiseptic and anti-microbial benefits of tea tree oils were being observed and recorded by A.R. Penfold, while in Italy Giovanni Gatti and Renato Cajola were investigating the psychological effects of essential oils. During World War II, an Army surgeon, Dr. Jean Valnet, utilized what he had learned from Gattefosse's work to treat soldiers wounded on the battlefield. He continued his medical practice after the war, incorporating essential oils into every phase. His definitive book, *The Practice of Aromatherapy*, was published in 1964 and is now available in English and widely read.

One of Valnet's students, biochemist Marguerite Maury, brought aromatherapy to Britain. Married to a French doctor and homeopath, Maury worked with essential oils medicinally and also researched their ability to penetrate the skin and to maintain youth. Thus, aromatherapy was adopted by beauty therapists qualified in massage techniques, which is why aromatherapy has been so closely connected with massage therapy. In her book *The Secret of Life and Youth*, Maury proposes the concept of an "individualized prescription"—a blend of essential oils that would harmonize the physical, psychological, and spiritual nature of the patient, thereby balancing and normalizing the whole person.

The list of significant contributors in the aromatherapy industry continued to grow and included the chemist Pierre Franchomme, Shirley Price, and Patricia Davis. However, it wasn't until 1977 with the publication of Robert Tisserand's *The Art of Aromatherapy*, one of the first English books on the subject, that the great interest in the medicinal properties of essential oils was sparked.

Today in Europe aromatherapy is incorporated into the traditional health care community, requiring professional licensure and prescriptions for oral use of aromatherapy.

In America, aromatherapy products are available through a variety of retail outlets. Book stores, libraries, and Internet sites are filled with aromatherapy information that describes the history, application, purported uses, and properties of essential oils.

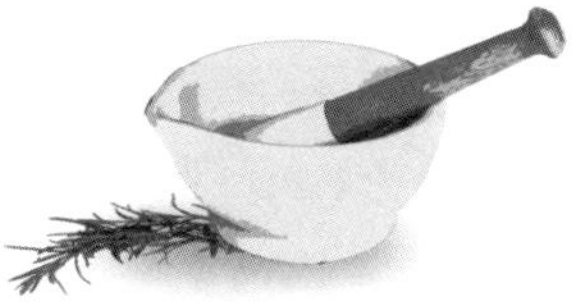

How Are Essential Oils Obtained?

One distinction that is important to recognize is that essential oils are quite different from herbal tinctures, flower remedies, or homeopathics.

- *Herbal tinctures* are concentrated extracts of herbs, usually using a mixture of water and alcohol to extract the constituents of the herb and act as a preservative. Tinctures are made over a four to six week period. The ratio of alcohol to water varies from one herb to another.

- *Flower essence* is a broad description for a liquid preparation that is created by immersing a flower into water and exposing the preparation to sunlight or heat. This infuses the preparation with healing properties that are derived from the life energy and spiritual elements contained in the flower. Flower remedies are products made from these essences. These can be Bach flower remedies (the original 38), or any of the newer flower remedies available today: Alaskan, Australian Bush, Perelandra, Green Hope Farms, Himalayan, Ancient Forrest, etc.

- *Homeopathic remedies* are diluted forms of natural substances made from plant, mineral, metal, and insect sources. The preparation of homeopathic remedies, known as potentization, consists of successive dilutions followed by shaking in ten hard strikes against an elastic body at each dilution stage. The vigorous agitation following each dilution is thought by believers in homeopathy to transfer some of the "spiritual essence" of the substance to the water. Homeopathy defines the potency of its remedies according to how diluted they are: the more diluted, the stronger it considers them.

Essential oils are derived from several different extraction methods:

- *Steam distillation*: This is the method most commonly used to obtain essential oils. Plant material is placed on a wire mesh in a large vat and then sealed. The water is then heated, and steam is passed through the plant material. The heat causes the glands in the plants to burst, releasing the volatile essential oils. The vaporized essences, along with steam and other substances, pass into a pipe through cooling tanks. This forces the vapors to return to liquid form as floral water plus essential oil. Since the essential oils are heavier than the floral water, the oil floats on top and is siphoned off. The floral waters (also called hydrosols, see sidebar) are also used in aromatherapy.

- *Carbon dioxide extraction:* Introduced in the early 1980s, this technology requires expensive, complicated equipment that uses carbon dioxide at very high pressures and extremely low temperatures. The higher cost for this type of extraction is worth it because this extraction method produces "cleaner" smelling oil, with a higher yield from the plant material.

- *Expression:* This process is commonly used for citrus fruits, where shred-

What are Hydrosols?

Also known as hydrolates, hydrolats, floral waters, or plant waters, hydrosols are the "water solution" that is produced during the steam distillation process for essential oils. Suzanne Catty considers hydrosols to be "The Next Aromatherapy."

Hydrosols contain the energy and water-soluble components of the original plant material being distilled. Easy to use for home, office, or travel, hydrosols are packaged in 120ml spray bottles. Refreshing, nurturing and healthy! Hydrosols do not have to be diluted or shaken prior to use and have endless uses and applications: as a spritzer, a room fragrance, in bath water, as a face toner, etc.

ding, scraping, squeezing, or pressing the plant material (usually the rind of the fruit) under cold pressure extracts the essential oils. It is also known as scarification. The storage life on these oils is shorter than that of distilled oil; they are best kept in a cool, dark place.

- *Solvent extraction:* This technique is used to extract materials that cannot be obtained by any other process. The plant material is immersed in a suitable solvent (acetone or any petroleum by-product), and the separation is performed either chemically or by distillation at specific temperatures that condense the oil but not the solvent. This is the least desirable method of extraction because these oils contain some traces of chemical solvents after the process.

- *Resinoids:* These are the solid or semi-solid substances obtained from the cut bark of trees or bushes. Hydrocarbons or alcohols are used to extract these natural gums or resins that contain heavy aromatic matter of low volatility. Resinoids are used as fixatives.

- *Concretes:* Similar to resinoids, except that plant material (i.e., leaves, flowers, roots, etc.) is used instead of the plant's resin. The solvent is then removed by vacuum distillation, leaving a mostly solid or semi-solid wax. Most concretes produce a salve-like/wax-like solid.

- *Absolutes:* Not true essential oils, absolutes are obtained from concretes that are treated with alcohol to separate the plant wax from the essential oil. A thickish, colored liquid remains after the alcohol is evaporated off under vacuum pressure. In some cases, a solvent such as benzyl benzoate may be added to improve fluidity.

- *Enfleurage:* Layers of plant material are placed over purified fat or wax over glass trays. Every day the flowers or plants are changed, until the fat is saturated with the plant extracts, then alcohol is added and removed to separate the essential oil from the fat. Similarly, maceration is used to extract essential oils from animal ingredients, vanilla, and iris. These materials are steeped into vats of oil until the scented parts dissolve. This process actually creates more of an "infused oil." The oil may be heated to speed up the process. Maceration is a long process, and in some cases, years.

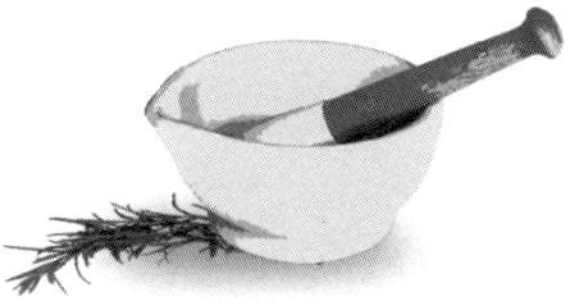

The Complexity of Essential Oils

Essential oils are complex substances. Being organic in nature, they contain carbon molecules that can form several dozen of atomic arrangements called functional groups. Some examples of functional groups include alcohols, aldehydes, esters, ketones, and phenols. These groups impart the medicinal properties of the oils. Therefore, just like pharmaceuticals that must not be adulterated, so the same is true for essential oils.

Many essential oil companies now provide gas chromatography and/or mass spectrometry to identify individual chemical components and to ensure the quality and therapeutic nature of the essential oil.

Some ways essential oils are adulterated include:

- Adding a chemical to the essential oil to "stretch" it.
- Adding oils from a cheaper plant.
- Adding a synthetic (chemical) aromatic substance, also known as "reconstituted."
- Removing some natural chemical constituents, thus altering the complexity of the essential oil.
- Diluting the essential oil with a carrier oil (such as jojoba) but not labeling it as such.

Why is it important to use pure essential oils? Synthetic oils, those made chemically in a laboratory and not directly extracted from the plant material, are not the dynamic, organic, life force of the plant. This is similar to synthetic medications, i.e., Sudafed® (pseudoephedrine,) and the plant from which this medication is derived, ephedra (ma huang). No chemical process can fully mirror a natural product. Synthetic substances may duplicate the smell, thickness, and color of the pure botanical, but it is the complex molecular components of each natural essential oil that determine its full therapeutic qualities. Additionally, synthetic substances can cause allergies and other possible side effects. Generally speaking, it is rare for a similar allergy to occur with a pure essential oil, unless the person is allergic to the plant material itself.

Likewise, the quality of essential oils is paramount. If an essential oil is to be therapeutic, it should be from the correct plant source, harvested at the right time, and grown under the correct conditions. The location, time of day, weather, and season dictate the best time to extract the essences. The quality, price, and intensity of the essential oils vary according to the variety of plant, the part of the plant used, the time of harvest, the richness of the soil, the quality and length of the cultivation methods, the process of distillation, and the reliability of the company providing the oils. The price of each essential oil is directly related to the amount of plant material needed for distillation, the country of origin, transportation costs, labor costs, and the difficulty with which they are extracted.

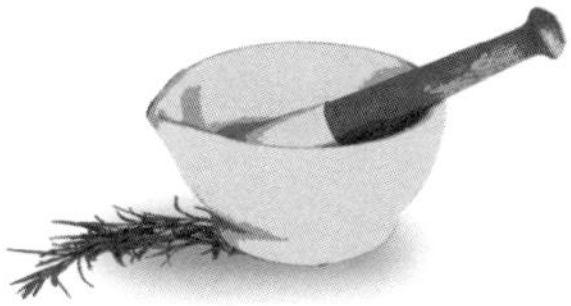

What Is the Difference between Essential Oils and Fragrance Oils?

Fragrance oils, also known as perfume oils, are synthetic. They are chemicals made in a laboratory. They are made to smell like essential oils derived from plant materials. The perfume industry uses synthetics extensively. Synthetic "essential oils" are usually a combination of derived chemicals that are mostly manmade and often produced from petroleum. Chemists take a natural compound to form the building blocks and then add a petroleum-derived substance.

Smell-wise, synthetics may sometimes smell "better," depending upon personal preference. Health-wise, they are fairly unhealthy. No chemical process does it better than nature. Synthetics do not consist of the same molecules that compose the natural substance. Natural oils get far better results and cause fewer allergic reactions and sensitivities.

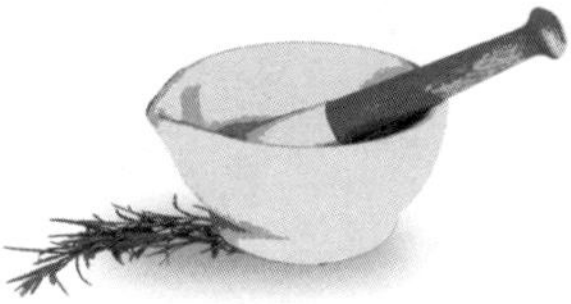

How Do Essential Oils Work?

Scientists do not know exactly how aromatherapy works, but put quite simply, essential oils work through the olfactory system. The sense of smell works on a subconscious level. Olfactory nerves conduct smell sensations to a part of the brain that also regulates behavioral mechanisms and sexual urges. The perfume industry grasped this fact early and has since used the concept of sexual stimulation through fragrances to sell its products.

The sense of smell is the most underappreciated and intangible sense, but it is 10,000 times more sensitive than that of taste. Humans are able to process up to 100,000 different smells. Aromas help us feel better and have a tremendous therapeutic effect on stress-related physical symptoms.

The olfactory system uses a "lock and key" mechanism to remember scents and create an individualized perception of aromas, preferences for different scents, and specific memory responses. The lock is the actual smell memory; the scent is the key which opens up the mind to the memory. The sense of smell has the longest recall of all the senses. Like smelling salts, different odors wake up the brain, evoking images and feelings associated with each smell. The sense of smell can be positive or negative, exhilarating or relaxing, calming or stimulating, warm or cold, vivid or vague.

Aromas enter through the nasal cavity. We receive odors through thousands of olfactory nerves in our nostrils that contain bundles of highly sensitive nerve cells on the membrane lining. The aromatic molecules of essential oils react with specific nerve receptors. Transmission of the aroma is sent directly to the limbic system, a part of the brain that stores responses to memory, pleasure, and emotions. Because the olfactory nerves are a direct extension of the limbic system in the brain itself, recognition of smell is relayed immediately, whereas the recognition of taste, sound, and touch is not as immediate.

Odor triggers the release of neurochemicals in the limbic system: *encephalin*, which reduces pain and creates a feeling of well being, *endorphins* that kill pain and induce sexual feeling, and *serotonin* which helps relax and calm. The brain not only interprets the aroma message by retrieving the memory of a past experience or creating a new memory response but also associates either a calming, balancing, or stimulating action response. Although vivid and indelibly etched in the limbic system's memory, scents are illusive, disappearing quickly.

When absorbed by the skin, inhaled, or ingested, essential oils are transported throughout the body to affect various organ functions. For example, oils can act as sedatives or stimulants, carminatives and digestive aids, or cause numerous other genuine physiological effects.

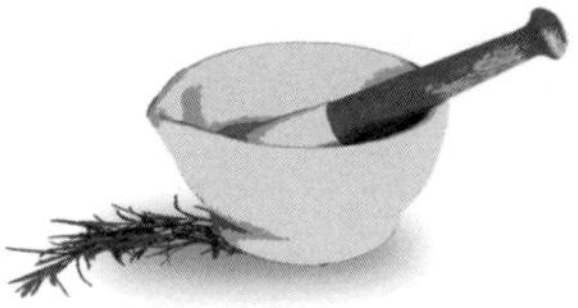

How to Use Essential Oils

Powerful and concentrated, essential oils have infinite uses: from health, body, and cosmetic uses to room scenting and housecleaning. They allow a great amount of versatility and creativity in their uses depending upon the specific oil, and your intended goal. You are only limited by the essential oil precautions, which are discussed later. Below are some of the most common ways to use essential oils:

For room diffusion:

- *Candles:* Light the candle and wait until some wax has melted, then add 1-2 drops to the warm wax. Essential oils are flammable so be careful not to get the oils on the wick. This method is not advocated for therapeutic use.

- *Diffusers:* Several different types of diffusers are available, especially developed for essential oils. Some are electric and some heated by candles. They can cover a room from 100 sq feet up to 1000 sq feet. Diffusers allow the essential oil molecules to become airborne into a fine mist and dispersed into the air. Electric diffusers that do not use heat for activation are the preferred method of room diffusion for therapeutic purposes. Other diffusers utilize a cotton pad on which to place the oils, and a fan that circulates the aroma on the pad.

- *Tabletop Diffusers:* Start with 5-10 drops on the porous part of the clay diffuser. Room temperature or sunlight allows the essential oil aromas to permeate the room.

- *Light Bulbs:* Always place oils on a cool bulb, not one that has been on for a while. Use light bulbs of 60 watts or lower. Place 1-2 drops on a light bulb ring, then turn on the light. If you do not have a light bulb ring, place 1-2 drops directly on the bulb, using caution not to allow the oils to drip down into the bulb attachment.

- *Humidifiers:* Add 3-6 drops to the water of the humidifier. If certain thick oils are used, this may present a problem for the filter system of your particular unit.

- *Room Sprays:* For every cup of water, use 5-10 drops of essential oil, and place in a clean plant sprayer or a mist spray bottle. Shake the mixture well before spraying and avoid wood furniture.

Externally:

The skin is the body's largest organ. When essential oils are applied externally, they are absorbed through the small blood vessels in the skin and carried to the muscles, joints, and blood stream, and then further to the tissues and organs. Just as allopathic drugs leave the body, so do essential oils—excreted through the kidneys and bladder and exhaled through the lungs. That is why it is so important to drink lots of water after a massage or a bath; it effectively helps the oils leave the body.

- *Bath for a full tub:* Run the bath water. A tepid bath (82-95°F or 28-35°C) is relaxing and sedative; a hot bath (95-102°F or 35-39°C) is restorative if it is short, but if it is very long can be enervating. Then add the essential oils. Remember to swish the water to disperse the essential oils thoroughly in the water so that the oils do not concentrate in one area, which may lead to skin irritations. Close the door to the bathroom so that the vapors are kept inside the room. Soak for at least 10 minutes, but no longer than 30 minutes. Relax and breathe deeply.

You can also:

- Mix 10-15 drops of essential oil in ½ cup bath salt mixture (let mixture set for one week before using, and shake frequently), or 1 cup Epsom salt.
- Mix 10-30 drops of essential oil in 15-30ml almond oil.
- Mix 10-30 drops in a small amount of grain alcohol or vodka.

● *For a foot bath:* Cut these proportions by 75%, to approximately 2-6 drops. Soak the feet for 10-20 minutes in a bowl of warm water.

● *Compress:* Add essential oils to a basin filled with hot or cold water (add 5-8 drops for application to a large body area and 2-4 drops for a smaller area). Agitate the water to disperse the oils evenly. Then place a handkerchief on top of the water, which will collect the floating oil. Gently squeeze out any excess water, and then apply the handkerchief to the affected area. Wrap a towel over the compress and leave it in place until the compress reaches body temperature, then repeat. Warm compresses are good for arthritic, menstrual, back, urinary, ear, tooth, or abdominal pains. Cold compresses are good for sunburn, headache, varicosities, and bruises.

● *Massage:* As a general rule, the essential oil content in massage oil should be 1-3%, depending on the particular indication. Some disorders require a stronger concentration, babies and children require a lower concentration, and pregnancy demands a weaker concentration.

Essential Oil	Base Oil
20-60 drops	100ml
7-25 drops	25ml
3-5 drops	5ml

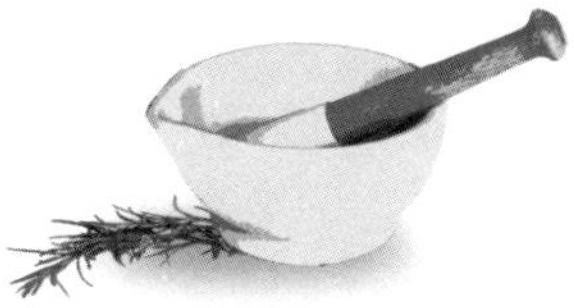

Essential Oil Safety and Precautions

With today's consumer revolution and the embrace of what is "natural," there is a misinterpretation that "natural" equates to "safe." However, essential oils are highly concentrated plant materials that possess strong medicinal qualities, and there are significant safety precautions. The best source of safety information is provided by the following professional organizations:

- According to their website, http://www.rifm.org, The Research Institute for Fragrance Materials (RIFM) evaluates and distributes scientific data on the safety assessment of fragrance raw materials found in perfumes, cosmetics, shampoos, creams, detergents, air fresheners, candles, and other personal and household products.

- The International Fragrance Association (IFRA), http://www.ifraorg.org, was founded in 1973 to represent the collective interests of the fragrance industry worldwide. The organization has established and seeks to preserve the self-regulatory practices of the international fragrance industry. This occurs through the development and implementation of a Code of Practice and safety standards utilized worldwide, with the final objective being to protect the consumer and the environment.

- The Fragrance Materials Association of the United States (FMA), http://www.fmafragrance.org, includes companies that invent and then manufacture mixtures of fragrance ingredients for use in a wide variety of products, including fine fragrances, shampoos, soaps, and detergents. FMA's activities involve legislative and regulatory work on the industry's behalf. It is closely coordinated with RIFM.

There are three basic types of adverse reactions that can occur when essential oils are applied to the skin:

- **Irritation:** Reactions from mild itch to burn when oil comes in contact with the skin. When the irritant is removed, the reaction starts healing.

- **Sensitization:** This is a more significant reaction than irritation causing reactions from mild itching to the extreme of anaphylactic shock. Anaphylaxis is the most severe allergic reaction. In anaphylaxis, immune chemicals, such as histamine, produce serious skin symptoms (hives, swelling) as well as severe breathing problems (swelling in the throat, narrowing of the lower airways, wheezing). They also produce a dramatic widening of the blood vessels, which results in a rapid, severe drop in blood pressure (shock). The incidence of anaphylaxis occurring in aromatherapy is unknown, but it is something for which to be alert. If an irritation, burning sensation, or irritable skin rash are noticed after first use, it may be that a sensitizing reaction is more likely to occur with repeated use of that essential oil or a chemically similar one.

- **Photosensitization/Phototoxicity:** This reaction occurs when a substance on the skin reacts with ultraviolet light. This includes ultraviolet light on cloudy days or in tanning salon equipment. This reaction can cause mild blotching to severe burning of the skin and can be very long lasting.

Skin Irritation and Sensitization

The best way to use essential oils topically is in the diluted form, with a few exceptions. Tea tree and lavender can be used directly on the skin in 1-2 drop quantities. Do a skin patch test if sensitivities are suspected.

To do a patch test correctly:

1. Clean and thoroughly dry the area to which the essential oil or blended product will be applied. Preferred areas are the inside elbow, the forearm, or behind the earlobe. If testing a blended massage oil, a small piece of gauze or cotton is needed.

2. For a massage oil, add 2 drops of the essential oil that is being tested in 1/2 teaspoonful of carrier oil. Apply a small amount to the skin and cover with gauze or cotton. Leave this area unwashed for 24 hours. If any redness or itching occurs, do not use that oil, as there may be an allergy to it.

3. If testing an undiluted essential oil, place a small drop on the skin and wait three to five minutes.

4. If there is any sign of stinging or skin irritation, use cream or vegetable oil to dilute, apply soap, wash with warm water. Repeat if necessary.

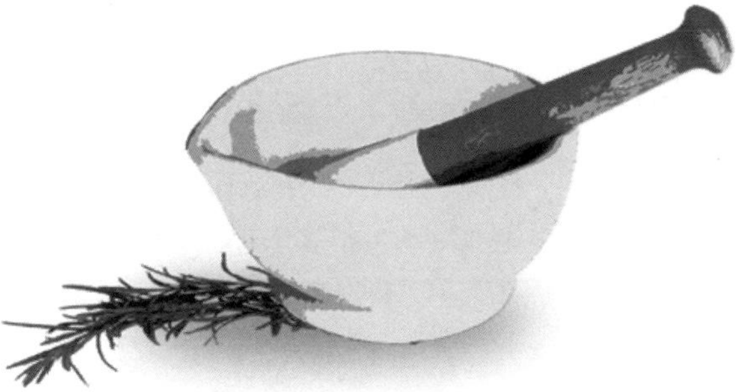

The following essential oils are IFRA Prohibited:

Common Name (*botanical name*)	**Rationale for IFRA Prohibition**
Cade oil crude (*juniperus oxycedrus*)	Carcinogen. Also known as prickly juniper or juniper tar.
Calamus oil (*acorus calamus*)	Some forms contain high levels of the carcinogen -asarone. Also known as sweet flag, myrtle flag, sweet rush, and sweet sedge.
Costus root oil, absolute & concrete (*saussurea costus*)	Sensitizing potential. Also known as kuth.
Elecampane oil (*inula helenium*)	Sensitizing potential. Also known as scabwort.
Fig leaf absolute (*ficus carica*)	Sensitizing and extreme phototoxic potential.
Horseradish (*armoracia rusticana*)	Toxic; irritant. Contains allyl isothiocynate.
Musk Ambrette (*hibiscus abelmoschus*)	Photosensitivity and neurotoxic effects.
Mustard oil (*brassica nigra*)	Toxic, irritant, high content (92% minimum) of allyl isothiocyanate. Also known as black mustard.
Sassafras oil (*sassafras albidum*)	Carcinogen—effectively banned by imposing a limit on the carcinogen safrole limit of 0.01% in perfumes. Examples of essential oils with high safrole content are sassafras officinale, ocotea cymbarum oil, ocotea pretiosa, and certain Camphor oils.
Savin oil (*juniperus sabina*)	High acute toxicity; juniperus phoenicea oil allowable.
Tea absolute (*thea sinensis, camellia sinensis*)	Sensitizing potential.
Verbena oil (*lippia citriodora*)	Sensitizing and extreme phototoxic potential.
Wormseed oil (*chenopodium ambroisoides*)	Acute oral toxicity affecting the liver and kidney.
Wormwood oil (*artemisia absinthium*)	Neurotoxicity; the active ingredient is thujone, which has convulsant and arbortifacient properties.

The following essential oils are IFRA Restricted and should only be used in appropriate concentrations or under the supervision of an experienced health care professional:

Common Name (***botanical name***)	**Rationale for IFRA Restriction**
Angelica root oil (*angelica archangelica*)	Phototoxic at 0.78%. For applications on areas of skin exposed to sunshine, excluding bath preparations, soaps, and other products that are washed off the skin, angelica root oil should be limited to 3.9% in the product.
Bergamot oil expressed (*citrus aurantium ssp. bergamia*)	Phototoxic at 0.4%, excluding bath preparations, soaps, and other products that are washed off the skin.
Bitter Orange oil (*citrus aurantium*)	Phototoxic at 1.25%.
Cassia oil (*cinnamomum cassia)*	Sensitizing potential at 0.2%.
Cinnamon bark oil (*cinnamomum zeylanicum*)	Sensitizing potential at 0.2%.
Cumin oil (*cuminum cyminum*)	Phototoxic at 0.4%, excluding bath preparations, soaps, and other products that are washed off the skin.
Grapefruit expressed (*citrus paradisi*)	Phototoxic at 4%, excluding bath preparations, soaps, and other products that are washed off the skin.
Lemon oil cold pressed (*citrus limonum*)	Phototoxic at 2%, excluding bath preparations, soaps, and other products that are washed off the skin.
Lime oil expressed (*citrus aurantifolia*)	Phototoxic at 0.7%, excluding bath preparations, soaps, and other products that are washed off the skin.
Oakmoss absolute and resinoid (*evernia prunastri*)	Sensitizing potential at 0.1%.
Opoponax solv extr or steam distil. (*commiphora erythraea var. glabrescens*)	Sensitizing potential at 0.6%.
Peru balsam extracts (*myroxylon pereirae*)	Sensitizing potential at 0.4%; distilled oil is allowable.
Pinaceae and isolates derived from the pinacea family, including pinus and abies genera	Sensitizing potential.

Common Name (***botanical name***)	**Rationale for IFRA Restriction**
Rue oil (*ruta graveolens*)	Phototoxic at 0.15%, excluding bath preparations, soaps, and other products that are washed off the skin. This recommendation is based on the fact that Rue oil is known to contain psoralenes.
Styrax resinoids, absolutes, and oils (*liquidamber orientalis, liquidamber styraciflua var. macrophylla*)	Sensitizing potential at 0.6%.
Tagete oil and absolute (*tagetes minuta, tagetes glandulifera, tagetes patula*)	Phototoxic at 0.01%, excluding bath preparations, soaps, and other products that are washed off the skin.
Treemoss absolute (*evernia furfuracea*)	Sensitizing potential at 0.1%.
Verbena absolute (*lippia citriodora*)	Sensitizing potential at 0.2%.

The following essential oils, although not officially IFRA Prohibited or Restricted, are considered toxic, and for safety reasons, should only be used under the supervision of an experienced health care professional:

Common Name (***botanical name***)	**Safety Issue**
Ajowan (*trachyspermum copticum*)	Due to 50% thymol content, ajowan is a mucous membrane and dermal irritant, and contraindicated in pregnancy.
Benzoin resinoid and oil (*styrax benzoin*)	Sensitizing potential.
Bitter Almond (*prunus amygdalus var. amara*)	Main constituent of oil is prussic acid (also known as cyanide) and even small amounts can be lethal.
Boldo (*peumus boldus*)	Although the essential oil demonstrated antimicrobial and fungicidal properties in a 1999 clinical study, boldo contains up to 40% asaridole, which is a documented liver toxin. Boldo also has demonstrated abortive and terratogenic properties.
Buchu (*barosma crenulata*)	Due to pulegone content, this oil is toxic and an abortifacient.

Common Name (***botanical name***)	**Safety Issue**
Camphor (*cinnamomum camphora*)	Brown and yellow camphor contain safrol that is toxic and carcinogenic. Although white camphor does not contain safrol, it can be irritating to the skin and must be highly diluted. Oral ingestion is toxic.
Copaiba (*copaifera officinalis*)	Sensitizing potential if the oil is old and oxidized.
Jaborandi (*pilocarpus jaborandi*)	The principal constituents are the three alkaloids, pilocarpine, isopilocarpine and pilocarpidine. Pilocarpine has shown to increase the rate of birth defects, can headaches and can irritate the stomach and cause vomiting and nausea. The plant may induce bradycardia. Jaborandi may induce dehydration due to excessive perspiration and urination.
Mugwort (*artemisia vulgaris*)	Due to high thujone content, this oil is an arbortifacient and a neurotoxin.
Pennyroyal (*mentha pulegium*)	Due to pulegone content, pennyroyal can cause death if ingested in large doses. In small doses, it produces acute liver and lung damage. The oil is toxic and an arbortifacient.
Southernwood (*artemisia abrotanum*)	Contains absinthol and thujone, which are abortifacients.
Tansy (*tanacetum vulgare*)	High in thujone, tansy can cause convulsions, and in small doses, can be lethal.
Thuja (*thuja occidentalis*)	Due to high thujone content, this oil is an arbortifacient and a neurotoxin.
Wintergreen (*gaultheria procumbens*)	Due to the high methyl salicylate (98%) content, wintergreen is toxic in excess and can cause liver and kidney damage, and should not be given to patients sensitive to aspirin or salicylates.

In addition to the oils listed above, there are other oils that may cause skin irritation to sensitive, inflamed, or allergic skin types. These oils must be highly diluted prior to use. They include:

- Allspice (*pimenta officinalis*)
- Aniseed (*pimpinella anisum*)
- Basil (*ocimum basilicum*)
- Bay (*laurus nobilis*)
- Birch (*betula lenta*)
- Black Pepper (*piper nigra*)
- Cajeput (*melaleuca cajeputi*)
- Cedarwood, Virginian/Red (*juniperus virginiana*)
- Cinnamon leaf (*cinnamomum zelyanicum*)
- Citronella (*cymbopogon nardus*)
- Clove bud, leaf, and stem (*syzygium aromatica*)
- Fennel (*foeniculum vulgare*)
- Fir needle, Siberian (*abies siberica*)
- Ginger (*zingiber officinalis*)
- Lemongrass (*cymbopogen citratus*)
- May Chang (*litsea cubeba*)
- Oregano (*origanum vulgare*)
- Oregano, Spanish (*thymus capitatus*)
- Parsley (*petroselinum sativum*)
- Pennyroyal, American (*hedeoma pulegioides*)
- Peppermint (*mentha piperita*)
- Rosemary (*rosmarinus officinalis*)
- Savory, Summer (*satureia hortensis*)
- Savory, Winter (*satureia montana*)
- Thyme, Red (*thymus vulgaris*)
- Thyme, Wild (*thymus serpyllum*)
- Tumeric (*curcuma domestica*)
- Ylang Ylang (in high concentrations) (*cananga odorata*)

Photosensitization/Phototoxicity:

Avoid exposure to ultraviolet rays for a minimum of four hours following application of photosensitive essential oils. In addition to the oils listed above, other essential oils that have the potential to be phototoxic oils include:

- Bay (*laurel nobilis*)
- Bitter Orange (*citrus aurantium*)
- Caraway (*carum carvi*)
- Cedarwood, Virginian (*juniperus virginiana*)
- Celery (*apium graveolens*)
- Cinnamon leaf (*cinnamomum zelyanicum*)
- Dill (*anethum graveolens*)
- Ginger (*zingiber officinale*)
- Khella (*ammi visnaga*)
- Lovage (*levisticum officinalis*)
- Mandarin (*citrus reticulata*)
- Melissa (*melissa officinalis*)
- Orange, Sweet (*citrus simensis*)
- Parsley (*petroselinum sativum*)
- St. John's Wort (*hypericum perforatum*)
- Tangerine (*citrus reticulata*)
- Yarrow (*achillea millefolium*)

In the United States, the Food and Drug Administration (FDA) reviews the evidence available about the risk of harm if a medication is used during pregnancy. Then it assigns each one to a "Pregnancy Category" (A, B, C, D, or X). Very few medications have been tested to the highest level of Category A, leaving the majority of medications in the unknown or caution status. Likewise, there is little published clinical research regarding essential oil use in pregnancy, and much of the information has been obtained using claimed adverse effects of internal herbal consumption. As a result, essential oil use in pregnancy should only be undertaken with the expert advise of a qualified health practitioner.

Essential oils that appear on the IFRA Prohibited and Restricted lists and the toxic lists should be completely avoided at any time. In pregnancy, essential oils that contain high percentages of natural chemicals that could make them a potential irritant should be avoided. In addition to the oils listed above, other essential oils to be extra cautious of during pregnancy include:

- Champaca (*michelia champaca*)
- Cornmint (*mentha arvensis*)
- Davana (*artemisia pallens*)
- Eucalyptus (*eucalyptus dives*)
- Lavender, Cotton (*santolina chamaecyparissus*)
- Lavender, Spike (*lavendula latifolia*)
- Marjoram, Spanish (*thymus mastichina*)
- Melissa (*melissa officinalis*)
- Tarragon (*artemisia dracunculus*)

Lastly, some essential oils may cross the placenta, and the effect on the fetus is unknown. Certain essential oils have emmenogogic actions that could theoretically induce a miscarriage or may be toxic to the fetus. Such oils should not be used in the first trimester of pregnancy. Thereafter, if necessary, a dilution of 1% is recommended for use. These include:

- Angelica (*angelica archangelica*)
- Anise (*pimpinella anisum*)
- Basil (*ocimum basilicum*)
- Cajeput (*melaleuca cajuputi*)
- Caraway (*carum carvi*)
- Cedarwood (*cedrus atlantica*)
- Celery (*apium graveolens*)
- Chamomile, German (*chamomilla recutita/matricaria recutita*)
- Chamomile, Roman (*anthemis nobilis*)
- Cinnamon leaf (*cinnamomum zelyanicum*)

- Citronella (*cymbopogon nardus*)
- Clary Sage (*salvia sclarea*)
- Clove bud, leaf, and stem (*syzygium aromatica*)
- Cypress (*cupressus sempervirens*)
- Fennel (*foeniculum vulgare*)
- Hyssop (*hyssop officinalis*)
- Jasmine (*jasminum officinalis*) (okay after 16 weeks)
- Juniper (*juniperus communis*)
- Lovage (*levisticum officinale*)
- Marjoram, Sweet (*organum majoriana*)
- Myrrh (*commiphora myrrha*)
- Nutmeg (*myristica fragrans*)
- Parsley (*petroselinum sativum*)
- Peppermint (*mentha piperita*)
- Rosemary (*rosemary officinalis*)
- Rose (*rosa damascena, rosa centifolia*)
- Sage (*salvia officinalis*)
- Thyme, White (*thymus vulgaris*)
- Vetiver (*vetiveria zizanioides*)
- Yarrow (*achillea millefolium*)

There is some anecdotal evidence that suggests some essential oils should be avoided with certain medical diagnosis. These essential oils are listed below. However, the clinical literature to demonstrate a contradiction with essential oils does not exist to any reportable extent. Proper usage of essential oils dictates that a single consistent oil be used for short term in low frequency, and if long-term therapy is necessary, that the essential oils be rotated during the course. Therefore, guidance from an experienced health care professional should be sought if the following concurrent illnesses exist:

Epilepsy

Many essential oils contain naturally occurring ketones that can easily penetrate the blood/brain barrier; the neurotoxic effects of these essential oils with high ketones have been documented.

- Anise (*pimpinella anisum*)
- Basil (*ocimum basilicum*)
- Camphor (*cinnamomum camphora*)
- Fennel (*foeniculum vulgare*)
- Hyssop (*hyssop officinalis*)
- Lavender, Spike (*lavendula latifolia*)
- Nutmeg (*myristica fragrans*)
- Parsley (*petroselinum sativum*)
- Rosemary (*rosmarinus officinalis*) (okay in small doses)
- Sage (*salvia officinalis*)

Glaucoma

There is some literature to suggest that the following essential oils can raise intraoccular pressure:

- Cypress (*cupressus sempervirens*)
- Hyssop (*hyssop officinalis*)
- Tarragon (*artemisia dracunculus*)
- Thyme (*thymus vulgarus*)

Kidney/Renal Disease

There is some literature to suggest that the following essential oils are nephrotoxic and/or can overstimulate the kidneys. This usually occurs when the oils are used in high doses for an excessive period of time.

- Bay (*laurel nobilis*)
- Cinnamon leaf (*cinnamomum zelyanicum*)
- Clove bud, leaf, and stem (*syzygium aromatica*)
- Coriander (*coriandrum sativum*)
- Juniper (*juniperus sabina*)
- Sandalwood (*santalum album*)

Liver Disease

There is some literature to suggest that essential oils with a high aldehyde content may cause the essential oils to build up in the liver. This has been seen following oral ingestion and in high dosages.

- Anise (*pimpinella anisum*)
- Basil (*ocimum basilicum*)
- Bay (*laurel nobilis*)
- Cinnamon leaf (*cinnamomum zelyanicum*)
- Clove bud, leaf, and stem (*syzygium aromatica*)
- Fennel (*foeniculum vulgare*)
- Nutmeg (*myristica fragrans*)
- Oregano (*oreganum vulgare*)
- Parsley (*petroselinum sativum*)
- Savory, Summer (*satureia hortensis*)
- Savory, Winter (*satureia montana*)
- Star Anise (*illicum verum*)
- Tarragon (*artemisia dracunculus*)
- Thyme (*thymus vulgarus*)

Cancer

In the US, between 30-40% of the public regularly uses some kind of alternative medicine practice. And 50% of cancer patients will turn to some type of unconventional practice during treatment.[1] Aromatherapy and massage are used frequently to help with cancer symptoms and overall well-being. Some precautions that need to be taken when using essential oils:

---

[1] Cassileth, B. R., & Chapman, C. C. (1996). "Alternative cancer medicine: A ten-year update." Cancer Investigation, 14, 396–404.

- Keep massage light and avoid deep massage techniques.
- Avoid massage near the lymph glands.
- Do not massage areas that have been treated with radiation.
- Do not massage areas that have skin cancers.

Essential oils have naturally occurring chemicals, albeit in minute quantities, that may be carcinogenic. However, when cancer is already present, care should be taken to avoid these oils. This list includes:

- Anise (*pimpinella anisum*)
- Basil (*ocimum basilicum*)
- Bay (*laurel nobilis*)
- Camphor (*cinnamomum camphora*)
- Cinnamon leaf (*cinnamomum zelyanicum*)
- Clove bud, leaf, and stem (*syzygium aromatica*)
- Fennel (*foeniculum vulgare*)
- Nutmeg (*myristica fragrans*)
- Star Anise (*illicum verum*)

Because of their high anethole[2] or citral[3] content, essential oils to avoid when an estrogen-dependent cancer is present are:

- Aniseed[2] (*pimpinella anisum*)
- Citronella[3] (*cymbopogon nardus*)
- Eucalyptus[3] (*eucalyptus globulus*)
- Fennel[2] (*foeniculum vulgare*)
- Lemongrass[3] (*cymbopogen citratus*)
- Melissa[3] (*melissa officinalis*)
- Star Anise[2] (*illicum verum*)
- Verbena[3] (*lippia citriodora*)

Skin cancers and melanomas:

- All citrus oils, including bergamot

---

[2] Albert-Puelo, M. (1980). "Fennel and anise as estrogenic agents." Journal of Ethnopharmacology. 2: 337-34.

[3] Geldof, A. (1992). "Estrogenic action of commonly used fragrant agent induces prostatic hyperplasia." Urological Research. 20:139-44.

Children respond well to aromatherapy if used safely. When making a massage oil for a child, dilute to one-third to one-half of what you would normally make for an adult, which for an adult is usually a 2% dilution. Children's bodies are smaller and their skins are also more sensitive, so using a maximum dilution of 1% would be considered safe. In addition to all the previously discussed essential oils, additional essential oils that that should not be used in children include:

- Anise (*pimpinella anisum*)
- Camphor (*cinnamomum camphora*)
- Eucalyptus (*eucalyptus dive and globules*)
- Lavender, Crested (*lavendula stoechas*)
- Lavender, Spike (*lavendula latifolia*)
- Peppermint (*mentha piperita*) if child is less than 30 months old
- Rosemary (*rosmarinus officinalis*) (camphor type-Spain and Croatia)
- Sage (*salvia officinalis*)
- Yarrow (*achillea millefolium*)

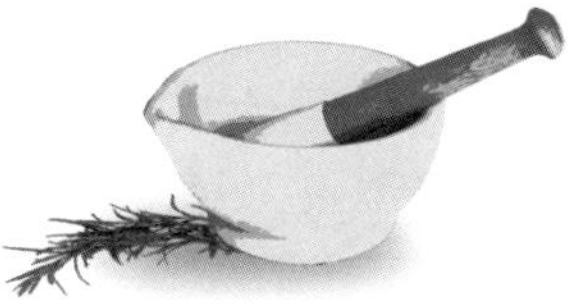

General Information and Care of your Essential Oils:

- Do not use on or near the eyes. If diluted essential oil accidentally gets into the eye, flush with clean warm water; if undiluted oils get is the eye, immediately flush with cold, full-fat milk or vegetable oil to dilute. If stinging is not alleviated, seek medical assistance.

- Do not take essential oils internally, unless under the guidance of a healthcare practitioner or professional aromatherapist. Because of the digestive process, oral use of essential oils is considered less effective than other methods of use.

- Keep all essential oils tightly capped, out of reach of children, and away from pets. When purchasing essential oils, ensure that a dropper top or orifice reducer is included in the bottle. This allows the essential oils to be measured out slowly, in drops.

- Essential oils should be labeled appropriately, with the common and botanical name of the plant. This will assist you in selecting the correct product.

- Do not place undiluted essential oils directly on skin. Certain oils can irritate the skin when applied neat (without dilution). Use extra care on broken or damaged skin.

- Keep away from light and heat sources. Essential oils are volatile and thus flammable.

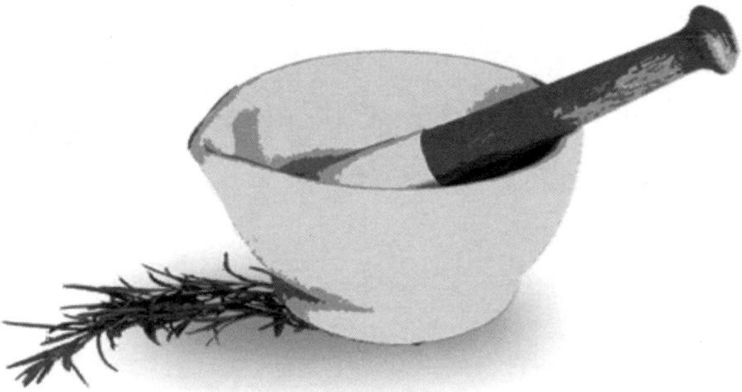

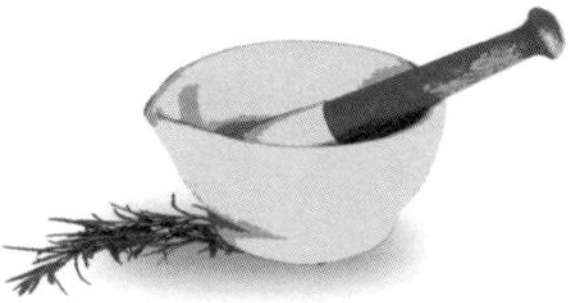

Aromatherapy Dilution

Massage

1% dilution: for children, the elderly, and pregnant women

- 1 tablespoon oil: 3 drops essential oil
- 1 ounce oil: 6 drops essential oil

2% dilution: for typical whole-body lotions and oils

- 1 tablespoon oil: 6 drops essential oil
- 1 ounce oil: 12 drops essential oil

2.5% dilution: average whole-body massage

- 1 tablespoon oil: 8-9 drops essential oil
- 1 ounce oil: 15 drops essential oil

4% dilution: for concentrated massage oils (local areas)

- 1 tablespoon oil: 12 drops essential oil
- 1 ounce oil: 24 drops essential oil

5% dilution: for concentrated massage oils (local areas)

- 1 tablespoon oil: 15 drops essential oil
- 1 ounce oil: 30 drops essential oil

Bath

- 5-8 drops per tub of water
- 1-2 drops in sitz bath
- 4-6 drops in foot bath

Inhalation

- 1-3 drops on a tissue or cotton pad
- 2-6 drops on a diffuser cartridge
- 1-3 drops on a clay personal or car diffuser
- 2-4 drops in the channel of a light ring
- 1-2 drops in a bowl or pot of hot water
- 2-4 drops in a humidifier

Compress

- 2 drops in a bowl of cold or warm water. Dip cotton cloth onto surface of water. Apply to affected area.

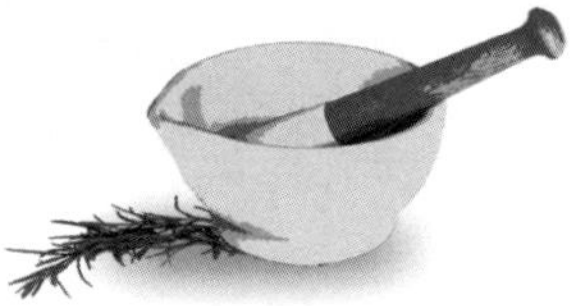

Aromatherapy Measurements

- 1 ml (cc) = 20-25 drops
- 1 teaspoon = 5 ml
- 1 tablespoon = 15ml
- 30ml = 1 ounce

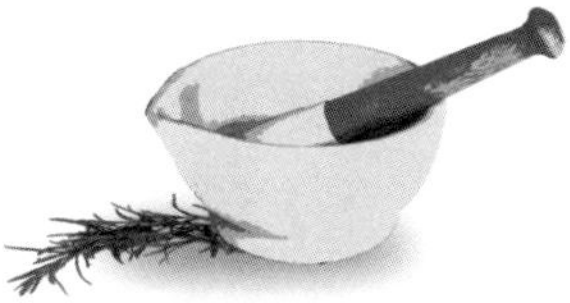

Essential Oils: Uses, Applications, Source, and Precautions

Essential oils in the chart below are listed alphabetically according to the common name. The botanical name (or scientific name) is provided to make the distinction of the appropriate plant in discussion. The botanical names have their origins in Latin and consist of two parts: the first is the genus to which the plant belongs and is always a noun; the second is the species name, which is commonly an adjective. Variety or cultivar names, if any, will follow and will not be italicized. The variety is a subgroup name in which the plant differs only slightly from the species. This further delineates a specific plant. It is important to know the botanical name of the plant so that the correct essential oil is used.

A description of the scent of the essential is given, followed by a brief summary of the most common traditional and/or documented uses of the essential oil. Blending information is provided from an aroma standpoint.

Essential oils are used in a variety of ways, depending upon the specific oil and condition. Possible applications are listed. Remember that topical application requires that the essential oils be diluted prior to use.

Like fine wine, plants cultivated for essential oil production have an optimal growing geography. The country of origin is important because the quality and quantity of essential oils vary with climate. Additionally, the chemical components of essential oils varies with the time of year, the time of day, the condition of the soil, the harvesting time, the altitude, etc. Hence, the same essential oil grown in different countries may smell differently and have slightly different therapeutic properties. The distillation is provided for information only.

Plants contain tiny sacs in or on the surface of the plant tissue that carry the essential oil. These sacs are found in the different part of the plants. In general, there is a correlation between the specific part of the plant from which the oil is extracted and its use on specific parts of the body. Essential oils obtained from different parts of the same plant can have different therapeutic qualities.

If using essential oils to blend perfumes, the "note" information is provided as a general guideline.

Although discussed at length earlier, precautions are listed again as a reminder.

This chart of essential oils is by no means meant to be complete or comprehensive; its sole purpose is to provide the reader "only the essentials" and serve as a quick reference guide.

Essential Oil Common Name (*botanical name*)	Aroma Traditional and/or documented uses Blending	Methods of Use	Country of Origin Distillation Method Part of the Plant Note	Precautions
Allspice (*pimento officinalis*)	• Spicy, warm, fragrant. • Improves circulation. Carminative; improves digestion. Purifying, helps in the reduction of cellulite. Calms the nerves, removes stress, and promotes a restful sleep. Vapors open the sinuses and breathing p assages. Mood uplifting. Loosens tight muscles, lessens pain. Aphrodisiac. • Blends well with frankincense, galbanum, ginger, lavender, lemon, lemongrass, nutmeg, orange, and pine.	Topical, room diffusion, inhalation, massage	• West Indies, Central America • Steam • Twigs, leaves and dried unripe berries • Middle to Top	Can be irritating to the skin.
Ambrette (*hibiscus abelmoschus*)	• Musky and sweet. • Calming, relieves nervous tension, and reduces stress. Mood uplifting. Lessens aches and pains. Healing and moisturizing to the skin. Aphrodisiac. • Blends well with clary sage, cypress, floral, wood and spice oils.	Topical, room diffusion, inhalation, bath, massage, perfume	• Ecuador • Steam • Seeds • Middle	Phototoxic.
Amyris (*amyris basamifera*)	• Musty, faintly woodsy. • Cooling, calming, reduces stress and tension; relieves anxiety, promotes a peaceful state. Helps to deepen the breathing. Reviving, improves mental clarity. Looses tight muscles. Used as a fixative to hold the scent of a fragrance; when used as a room fragrance, makes a less expensive alternative to Sandalwood. • Blends well with citronella, lavender, oakmoss, and other wood oils.	Topical, room diffusion, bath, inhalation, massage, bath, perfume	• West Indies • Steam • Wood chips • Middle to Base	

Essential Oil Common Name (*botanical name*)	Aroma Traditional and/or documented uses Blending	Methods of Use	Country of Origin Distillation Method Part of the Plant Note	Precautions
Angelica (*angelica archangelica*)	• Sweet, musky, earthy, and herbal with a spicy undertone. • The herb is included in the famous Chartreuse and Benedictine liqueur. Relieves nervous exhaustion and stress and revitalizes the mind. Useful for dull, congested skin and psoriasis. Invigorates the lymphatic system and used for general detoxification. Stimulates the appetite, and is useful for flatulence and indigestion. Said to control uric acid and may be beneficial to rheumatic conditions, arthritis, gout, and sciatica. • Blends well with well with basil, bergamot, cedarwood, chamomile, citruses, clary sage, coriander, frankincense, geranium, grapefruit, lavender, lemon, mandarin, patchouli, and vetiver.	Topical, room diffusion, bath, inhalation, massage	• Europe • Steam • Rhizome, seed, and herb • Top to Middle	Phototoxic. Avoid during pregnancy and diabetes.
Anise Seed (Aniseed, Green Anise) (*pimpinella anisum*)	• Sweet and spicy, warming and stimulating. • Antispasmodic, sedative. Restores equilibrium to autonomic nervous system. Has estrogen-mimicking effects and can be used for amenorrhea. Carminative. Calming and relaxing and promotes a restful sleep. • Blends well with black pepper, coriander, cumin, fennel, and citrus oils.	Topical, bath, inhalation, room diffusion, massage	• Central and South America, Indonesia, India • Steam • Whole plant • Top	Avoid in children less than 10 years old and in pregnancy. Avoid in women with breast cancer. Avoid in epilepsy.

Anise, Star (*illicium verum*)	• Warm, sweet, and licorice-like. • Carminative, stimulant, diuretic. Fights cough and bronchitis by loosening phlegm. It has an antispasmodic effect on the intestines, thus relieving cramps. • Blends well with basil, fennel, and citrus oils.	Inhalation, room diffusion, massage (highly diluted)	• Southern China and Vietnam • Steam • Pericarp • Top	
Arina (Iary) (*psiadia altissima*)	• Sharp, herbaceous, spicy undertones. • Warming, increases circulation. Opens breathing. Calming, reduces stress, relaxing to the mind. Looses tight muscles. Promotes sleep and encourages dreaming. May be useful for toothache, itching, and wound healing. • Blends well with citrus and other wood oils.	Topical, bath, inhalation, room diffusion, massage	• Madagascar • Steam • Whole plant • Middle	
Balsam Peru (*myroxylon pereirae*)	• Warm, vanilla-sweet, fresh, earthy, balsamic scent. • Used as a fixative and fragrance component in soaps, detergents, creams, lotions and perfumes. Warming and comforting, helpful for nervous tension and stress. An anti-inflammatory and anti-infectant, useful for respiratory disorders such as asthma, chronic cough, and bronchitis. May relieve dry, chapped skin, eczema, rashes, scabies, sores, and wounds. • Blends well with florals, patchouli, petitgrain, sandalwood, and spices.	Topical, bath, inhalation, room diffusion, massage, perfume	• El Salvador • Resin extraction • Bark • Base	

Essential Oil Common Name (*botanical name*)	Aroma Traditional and/or documented uses Blending	Methods of Use	Country of Origin Distillation Method Part of the Plant Note	Precautions
Balsam Tolu (*myroxylon balsamum*)	• Warm, pleasantly sweet, and fresh scent. • Used as a fixative and deodorant. Works primarily on the respiratory mucous membranes; good for chronic catarrh and non-inflammatory chest complaints, laryngitis, and croup. Helpful for cracked nipples, lips, cuts, and bedsores. • Blends well with cedarwood, labdanum, neroli, patchouli, sandalwood, and ylang ylang.	Topical, bath, inhalation, room diffusion, massage, perfume	• Venezuela • Resin extraction • Bark • Base	
Basil (*ocimum basilicum*)	• A wonderful fresh and sweet scent, reminiscent of anise. • Stimulant; uplifting and energizing for mental exhaustion, anxiety, stress, and fatigue. Antispasmodic, anti-inflammatory, nervous system regulator. Digestive tonic, carminitive, liver stimulant, and neurotonic. • Blends well with citrus, geranium, lavender.	Topical, room diffusion, inhalation, massage	• Europe, US, Madagascar, France • Steam • Flowering tops and leaves • Top	Avoid in pregnancy and in children.
Bay Laurel (*laurus nobilis*)	• Spicy, fresh, and strong. • Expectorant, mucolytic, viricide, and antifungal. Effective against candida (albicans, tropicalis, and pseudo-tropicalis) and a broad range of pathogenic bacteria. Stimulates lymph and blood circulation. Used as a scalp rub, it refreshes and stimulates hair follicles. Analgesic, antiseptic, antispasmodic, astringent, diuretic, and hepatic stimulant. Good for muscular pain, neuralgia, and general fatigue. • Blends well with cedarwood, citrus, coriander, cypress, fir, juniper, lavender, pine, rosemary, and spice oils.	Topical, room diffusion, massage, inhalation	• Mediterranean area, Europe, US • Steam • Leaves • Middle to Top	Use sparingly for external applications to avoid potential sensitization.

Benzoin (*styrax benzoin*)	• Vanilla-like aroma. • Warming and calming effect on tension and stress. Eases exhausted emotional and psychic states. Tonic to the lungs; beneficial action for bronchitis, asthma, coughs, colds, laryngitis, and sore throats. Calming effect on stomach, aiding digestion. Strengthens pancreas and controls blood sugar. Used as a fixative in perfume blends. • Blends well with copaiba, frankincense, jasmine, lemon, rose, sandalwood, and spice oils.	Topical, massage, perfume	• Java, Sumatra, Thailand • Steam • Resin • Base	
Bergamot (*citrus bergamia*)	• Light, floral, and fruity. • Refreshing, uplifting. Antidepressant, soothing, calming, balancing. Useful for nervousness, agitation, insomnia, and emotional crisis. Helps calm hyperactivity and anxiety. Antiseptic, antispasmodic, and stomachic. • Blends well with coriander and all florals.	Topical, bath, room diffusion, inhalation, massage	• Ivory Coast, Southern Italy, Guinea • Expressed • Rind • Top	Photosensitizing.

Essential Oil Common Name (*botanical name*)	Aroma Traditional and/or documented uses Blending	Methods of Use	Country of Origin Distillation Method Part of the Plant Note	Precautions
Bergamot mint (*mentha citrata*)	• Fresh, minty, citrusy; softer than peppermint. • Tonifying for nervous exhaustion. Strengthens weakened ovaries, is a male sexual tonic. A hepatic and pancreatic stimulant. Useful for intestinal spasm. • Blends well with benzoin, eucalyptus, lavender, lemon, other mints, and rosemary.	Topical, room diffusion, inhalation, massage	• Mediterranean, US • Steam • Leaves and flowering tops • Top	Photosensitizing.
Birch, Sweet Yellow (*betula alleghaniensis*)	• Aromatic, wintergreen. • Very specific use as a counterirritant in anti-arthritic/neuralgic ointments and analgesic balms. Good as an antispasmodic for overworked muscles, sprains, and painful joints. Helpful in cases of poor circulation, accumulation of toxins in the muscles, edema, and cellulite. • Blends well with cardamom, chamomile, frankincense, ginger, lavender, lemon, and orange.	Topical, massage	• Canada, USA • Steam • Bark • Middle to Top	Always dilute to avoid skin irritation. Avoid in pregnancy and epilepsy.
Birch, Sweet (*betula lenta*)	• Minty and sharp, similar to wintergreen. • Invigorating. A lymphatic cleanser, stimulates sweat glands aiding the body in releasing harmful toxins. Increases the flow of urine. Eliminates uric acid in joints. Analgesic; dulls pain by delaying the pain message to the CNS. Good anti-inflammatory and antispasmodic for overworked muscles, painful joints, and arthritis. • Blends well with other balsamic and woody oils.	Topical, room diffusion, inhalation, massage	• Russia, Germany • Tree bark • Steam • Middle to Top	Always dilute to avoid skin irritation. Avoid in pregnancy and epilepsy.

Birch, White (*betula alba*)	• Smoky, woody-green balsamic scent. • Purifying; helps in the reduction of cellulite. Relieves achy, tense, and sore muscles, reduces inflammation, lessens pain, especially in the joints. • Blends well with other balsamic and woody oils.	Massage	• North America • Steam • Buds and bark • Middle to Base	Avoid in pregnancy.
Bitter Almond (*prunus dulcis var. amara*)	• Sweet, cherry scent. • Used in the preparation of many beauty products, to hydrate skin, smooth wrinkles, dermatitis or skin burns.	Topical	• Asia, Middle East, Italy, Spain • Maceration, Steam • Kernels • Middle	Not recommended for aromatherapy or home use. Use rectified, as a preservative.
Bitter Orange (*citrus aurantium ssp. amara*)	• Bitter, fresh, and sweet. • Used as an analgesic and digestive tonic to help relieve nausea and soothe stomach disturbances such as indigestion, flatulence, and bloating. Antifungal and astringent. Anti-inflammatory, helpful in muscle and rheumatic pain and gout. • Blends well with cinnamon, clary sage, labdanum, lavender, lavendin, lemon, myrrh, oakmoss, and rosemary.	Topical, room diffusion, massage	• Mediterranean • Cold Pressed • Dried or almost ripe outer peel • Top	Phototoxic
Black Pepper (*piper nigrum*)	• Warm, fresh, and spicy. • Analgesic; increases circulation and is good for rheumatism and muscular aches. Aphrodisiac and sexual tonic. Useful for sluggish liver, pancreas, and digestion. • Blends well with florals, frankincense, lavender, and other spices.	Topical, massage, perfume	• India, Brazil, Southeast Asia • Steam • Fruit • Middle	Always dilute to avoid skin irritation. Use with caution in pregnancy.

Essential Oil Common Name (*botanical name*)	Aroma Traditional and/or documented uses Blending	Methods of Use	Country of Origin Distillation Method Part of the Plant Note	Precautions
Black Spruce (*picea mariana*)	• Fresh, woody, earthy, and sweet. • Bronchial decongestant. Tonic for endocrine system, especially useful in hyperthyroidism and adrenal exhaustion. Helps the body adapt to stress. • Blends well with citruses and other wood oils.	Topical, room diffusion, bath, inhalation, massage	• North America • Steam • Bark and branches • Middle	Use with caution in pregnancy.
Blue Cypress (*callitris intratropica*)	• Warm, woodsy with earthy undertones. • Anti-inflammatory; good for allergic hives, arthritis, and general joint pain and swelling. Soothes diaper rash. Antiviral; useful for common warts, cold sores, and shingles. • Blends well with citruses, florals, green scents, lemon myrtle, and lavender.	Topical, room diffusion, massage, bath, perfumery	• Australia • Steam • Heartwood • Base	
Buddha Wood (Desert Rosewood) (*eremophilla mitchelli*)	• Sweet, long lasting woody note. • Relaxing, spiritually connecting. Useful for pain relief of sore muscles and joints. Good for blending as a fixative, especially in men's toiletries. • Blends well with other wood and citrus oils.	Room diffusion, massage, perfumery	• Australia • Steam • Heartwood • Base	
Cajeput (*melaleuca leucandendron*) (*melaleuca cajeputi*)	• Medicinal and fruity scent. • Antibacterial, antispasmodic, analgesic. Stimulating, clears thought. Eases chronic pulmonary disease and helpful for asthma. Antiseptic effect on urinary system. Beneficial for acne and psoriasis. • Blends well with birch, eucalyptus, juniper, and peppermint.	Topical, bath, room diffusion, inhalation, massage	• Australia • Steam • Leaves and Buds • Medium	Avoid in pregnancy.

Camphor, White (*cinnamomum camphora*)	• Clear, strong, and fresh scent. • A counterirritant in rheumatism, muscular pains, sprains, and arthritis. Positive effect for bronchitis, coughs, colds, fever, flu, and infectious diseases. Useful in acne. Good in a spritzer to repel insects such as flies and moths. • Blends well with basil, cajuput, chamomile, lavender, and melissa.	Inhalation, room diffusion, topical if diluted	• China • Steam • Chipped Wood • Top	Always dilute to avoid skin irritation. Use with caution in pregnancy. Can over stimulate the adrenal glands.
Capsicum (*capsicum frutescens*)	• Hot and spicy. • Used primarily as a strong rubefacient to stimulate the circulation, aiding the removal of waste products and increasing the flow of nutrients to the tissues. Relieves painful muscle spasms, and is useful for arthritis, general muscle soreness, and diabetic neuropathy. Applied to the skin it desensitizes nerve endings and is used as a local anesthetic.	Topical, massage	• Mexico, India, China • Oleoresin • Fruit • Base	Always dilute to avoid skin irritation. Contact with eyes and mucous membranes should be avoided.
Caraway (*carum carvi*)	• Strong, warm, sweet, and spicy scent. • Antispasmodic, carminative; useful in gastric spasm and flatulence, Nervous tonic, eases mental strain and fatigue. Increases urine and flushes out toxins. Liver tonic. Mucolytic, helpful for bronchitis. Diminishes vertigo. • Blends well with cinnamon and other spices.	Topical, bath, room diffusion, massage	• Europe, Asia • Steam • Seeds • Middle	In excessive doses, it is neurotoxic and abortive. Use with caution in pregnancy.

Essential Oil Common Name (*botanical name*)	**Aroma Traditional and/or documented uses Blending**	**Methods of Use**	**Country of Origin Distillation Method Part of the Plant Note**	**Precautions**
Cardamom (*elettera cardamomum*)	• Sweet, spicy, balsamic, and warming. • A carminative; activates neurotransmitters that stimulate the digestive tract. Antispasmodic; useful for strong intestinal cramps and constipation. Helpful for the common cold and bronchial ailments. Relaxant; good for mental fatigue. Used as an exotic addition to perfumes. • Blends well with cedarwood, frankincense, orange, neroli, rose, and ylang ylang.	Topical, room diffusion, bath, inhalation, massage, perfume	• Guatemala, India • Steam • Seeds • Middle	
Carrot Seed (*daucus carota*)	• Earthy, sweet, and fruity. • Used in convalescence to regenerate the liver. Displays a revitalizing effect on the skin suffering from a lack of tone; useful for revitalizing and regenerating mature or damaged skin. • Blends well with citruses, fennel, frankincense, geranium, and spice oils.	Topical, bath, inhalation, massage	• Europe, Asia, North Africa, France • Solvent extracted, CO2 • Seed • Middle	
Cassia (*cinnamomun camphora*)	• Strong, spicy, woody scent. • Mood uplifting, reviving, helps to relieve fatigue. Disinfectant. Can assist with fevers, colds, flu, low vitality, and chills. • Blends well with balsams, mandarin, orange, spices, and ylang ylang.	Room diffusion	• Asia • Steam • Young leaves, twigs, and bark • Middle	"Hot" oil; can cause skin irritation. Not advisable for topical application. Avoid in pregnancy.

Cedarwood (*cedrus atlantica*)	• Woody-fruity scent. • Soothing and grounding qualities. Mucolytic. Counteracts water and lipid retention; useful against cellulite. Powerful stimulant on the circulatory system and metabolism. Lymph tonic. Antiseptic; useful in respiratory and urinary infections. • Blends well with bergamot, cypress, jasmine, juniper, neroli, other wood oils, and ylang ylang.	Topical, bath, inhalation, room diffusion, massage	• Africa, North America • Steam • Wood • Base	Avoid in children less than 10 years old and in pregnancy.
Cedarwood, Himalayan (*cedrus deodora*)	• Warm, dry, woody, and slightly smoky. • Uplifting and toning. Comforting and reviving. A strong antiseptic and astringent. Relieves respiratory congestion. Good for oily skin and scalp problems. Considered an aphrodisiac in that it is grounding and inspiring at the same time. An effective bug repellent. Acts as a fixative in perfumery. • Blends well with basil, bergamot, eucalyptus, chamomile, citruses, clary sage, cypress, frankincense, jasmine, rosemary, rosewood, sandalwood, vetiver, and ylang ylang.	Topical, bath, room diffusion, massage, inhalation	• India, Western Himalayas • Steam • Bark • Base	Use with caution in pregnancy.
Cedarwood, Red (*juniperus virginiana*)	• Warm, soft, and woody. It strongly resembles the aroma of cedar chests and closets. • Calming, relieves anxiety and nervous tension, and promotes a restful sleep. Good for meditation. Circulatory decongestant, helpful for varicose veins, and hemorrhoids. • Blends well with bergamot, cypress, jasmine, juniper, neroli, rosemary, other wood oils, and ylang ylang.	Topical, bath, room diffusion, massage, inhalation	• North America • Steam • Sawdust and wood Chips of the red cedar tree • Base	Avoid in pregnancy.

Essential Oil Common Name (*botanical name*)	Aroma Traditional and/or documented uses Blending	Methods of Use	Country of Origin Distillation Method Part of the Plant Note	Precautions
Cedarwood (*chamaecyparis lawsoniana*)	• Sweet, woody, and herbal scent. • Very gentle on the body and skin and useful for minor skin irritations, rashes, cuts, and abrasions. Antibacterial, antiviral, and antifungal. Has a relaxing and decongestant effect and is excellent for sinus and chest congestion, respiratory conditions, and breathing problems like asthma. Relieves tension and stress, and can be used as a general and nerve tonic. • Blends well with cypress, juniper, lavender, pine, and sandalwood.	Topical, bath, room diffusion, massage, inhalation	• USA • Steam • Sawdust • Base	
Celery (*apium graveolens*)	• Herbal, fresh, and slightly spicy. • Extensively used as a flavoring agent in foods, in alcoholic and soft drinks, and as a fragrance component in soaps, detergents, cosmetics, and perfumes. Useful in arthritis, helping to detoxify the body and improve the circulation of blood to the muscles and joints. Known to increase the elimination of uric acid and is useful for gout, neuralgia, and rheumatism. Mild diuretic and antiseptic, useful for cystitis, bladder, and kidney complaints. • Blends with lavender, lovage, oakmoss, opopanax, lovage, pine, other spices, and tea tree.	Topical, inhalation, massage	• India, Europe • Steam • Seeds • Top to Middle	May cause photodermatitis. Avoid in pregnancy.

Chamomile, Moroccan (Blue Tansy) (*tanacetum annum*)	• Sweet scent and deep blue in color, due to its high chamazulene content. • Anti-inflammatory, antihistamine, and antiallergenic properties. Useful for sunburns, inflamed, or damaged skin. Antibacterial. Neurotonic; good for nervous depression. Useful in hay fever, asthma, hives, and nonspecific rashes. • Blends well with citruses, clary sage, geranium, and patchouli.	Topical, bath, room diffusion, massage	• France, England, Spain, Egypt, Belgium, Germany, Italy, Hungary • Steam • Flowers • Middle	Maximum concentration of 5% works best.
Chamomile, German (*matricaria recutita*) (*matricaria chamomilla*)	• Heavy, floral, and pungent. One of the most reliable anti-inflammatory agents. High in alpha bisabolol and chamazulene, it is useful for soothing eczema, psoriasis, and itchy, dry, red, inflamed, and sensitive skin problems. Calms gastric and stomach ulcers. Analgesic for muscle pain and spasms, arthritis, and rheumatism. Good for boils or abscesses in a hot compress. • Blends well with citruses, clary sage, geranium, patchouli, and rose.	Topical, bath, room diffusion, inhalation, massage	• France, England, Spain, Hungary, South America, Belgium, Germany, Italy • Steam • Flowers • Middle	
Chamomile, Roman (*anthemis nobilis*)	• Sweet, fresh, apple-like fragrance. • Powerful antispasmodic, anti-inflammatory, and muscle relaxant. Good for muscle spasms and rheumatism. An emergency remedy during asthma attacks (rubbed on solar plexus, wrists, and temples.). Relieves insomnia, nervous depression, and nervous shock. Used for hyperactivity, to calm restless children, and for teething pain. • Blends well with citruses, geranium, lavender, patchouli, and rose.	Topical, bath, room diffusion, inhalation, massage	• France, England, Spain, Bulgaria, Belgium, Germany, Italy, Hungary • Steam • Flowers • Middle	

Essential Oil Common Name (*botanical name*)	Aroma Traditional and/or documented uses Blending	Methods of Use	Country of Origin Distillation Method Part of the Plant Note	Precautions
Champaca (*michelia alba*)	• Floral and spicy. • Warming, calming, promotes a peaceful state, reduces stress, useful in meditation. Mood uplifting, euphoric. Aphrodisiac. Purifying to the tissues. Helps easy breathing. • Blends well with citruses, other florals, and wood oils.	Topical, bath, inhalation, massage, perfumery	• Asia, India • Steam • Flowers and leaves • Middle	Avoid in pregnancy.
Cinnamon (*cinnamomum zeylanicum*)	• Sharp, spicy, stimulating, and warming. • Broadly effective antiseptic: effective against 98% of all Gram + and Gram - pathogens. Effective against yeasts, candida (albicans, tropicalis, and pseudo-tropicalis), and fungi, including aspergillus. Antiparasitic and prevents fermentation in the intestines. Effective against diarrhea, colitis, amoebic dysentery, bacterial cystitis, and UTI with e. coli. A muscle warmer and analgesic, useful for general aches and pains. • Blends well with balsams, mandarin, orange, and ylang ylang.	Topical, room diffusion, inhalation, massage	• Asia, Madagascar, India • Steam • Bark and leaves • Middle	Bark is irritating to the skin, and best used either highly diluted or in diffuser blends. Potential skin irritant and sensitizing agent. Not to be used with children less than 12 years old. Avoid in pregnancy.
Citronella (*cymbopogon nardus*)	• Lemony and tarty. • Antispasmodic, anti-inflammatory. Classically used as an insect repellent. Antiseptic, antispasmodic. Specific for oily skin and excessive perspiration. A room deodorizer. • Blends well with bergamot, cedarwood, geranium, lemon, orange, and pine.	Topical, room diffusion, inhalation, massage	• Asia, Madagascar, South America • Steam • Grass • Top	May be a skin irritant in strong dilutions. Photosensitizing.

Clary Sage (*salvia sclarea*)	• Musky and herbaceous. • Antistress, antifungal, spasmolytic. Contains a hormone-like molecule similar to estrogen, making it useful for PMS, dysmenorrhea, oligomenorrhea, and menopausal stress symptoms. Calming yet uplifting, relaxing, and euphoric; useful for nervous tension. Balancing for dry, oily, or inflamed skin. • Blends well with bergamot, jasmine, lavender, mandarin, and orange.	Topical, bath, room diffusion, inhalation, massage	• Russia, Morocco, Southern France, US, Syria • Steam • Flowering tops and foliage • Middle to Base	May cause complications with conditions sensitive to estrogen. Very relaxing; caution before driving. Use in small amounts. Use with caution in pregnancy.
Clove Bud (*eugenia caryophyllata*)	• Spicy, warming, and stimulating. • Antiviral, antifungal, antiparasitic, broad-spectrum antibacterial; used for warts, colds, flus, and other respiratory conditions. Traditionally used in tiny doses as a local anesthetic for toothache (Tappe Paste), for the high eugenol content. Good for exhaustion and stress. Helpful for muscle pain and rheumatism. • Blends well with citruses, clary sage, rosemary, other spices, and ylang ylang.	Topical, room diffusion, inhalation, massage	• Asia • Steam • Buds, leaves, stems • Middle	Potential skin irritant and sensitizing agent. Use in less than 1% dilution. Oil from bud is less irritating than leaves. Large amounts raise blood pressure. Avoid use in children. Use with caution in pregnancy.
Combava (*citrus hystrix*)	• Lemony, sweet, fresh, tangy, and somewhat exotic scent. • Useful for muscle aches and pain, sprains, arthritis, and rheumatic conditions. Helpful for anxiety, stress, and insomnia. • Blends wells with basil, citruses, clary sage, clove, florals, frankincense, geranium, marjoram, neroli, palmarosa, patchouli, sandalwood, and vetiver.	Topical, bath, room diffusion, inhalation, massage, perfume	• Madagascar • Steam • Leaves and twigs • Top to middle	

Essential Oil Common Name (*botanical name*)	**Aroma Traditional and/or documented uses Blending**	**Methods of Use**	**Country of Origin Distillation Method Part of the Plant Note**	**Precautions**
Copaiba (*copaifera officinalis*)	• Sweet and woody. • Warming, improves circulation. Calming; enhances relaxation and restful sleep and reduces stress. Mood uplifting, improves mental clarity and alertness. Useful for mediation. Anti-inflammatory, antibacterial, astringent. Healing and moisturizing for the skin. Good as a fixative for perfumes. • Blends well with other woods, geranium, and citrus oils.	Topical, bath, room diffusion, inhalation, massage, perfume	• Brazil, Columbia, Peru, Venezuela • Steam • Resin • Base	
Coriander (*coriandrum sativum*)	• Herbal, woodsy, and sweet. • Relaxing, antiseptic, strengthening. Can cause a mild feeling of euphoria. Uplifting, refreshing, and may help memory. Useful for dyspepsia, promoting digestion, and relieving stomach cramps. Used as a replacement for endangered rosewood. • Blends well with bergamot, citruses, clary sage, fir needle, ginger, jasmine, neroli, and spice oils.	Topical, bath, room diffusion, inhalation, massage	• Russia, India, Italy, Morocco, US • Steam • Seeds of ripe fruits and leaves • Middle	Use with caution in pregnancy.
Cornmint (*mentha arvensis*)	• Strong, fresh, nutty aroma. • Similar uses as peppermint, but contains a greater amount of menthol (60-80%.) Used for relief of headaches caused by nervousness. Also used for rheumatic pain, indigestion, nausea, sore throat, diarrhea, and colds. • Blends well with benzoin, eucalyptus, lavender, lemon, marjoram, other mints, and rosemary.	Room diffusion, inhalation, massage if highly diluted	• China • Steam • Flowering herb • Top	Must be diluted; is a dermal irritant.

Cumin (*cumimum cyminum*)	• Warm, soft, musky scent. • Helpful for chronic viral diseases. CNS relaxant. Good muscular spasmolytic. Relieves gastric pain and flatulence. Highly stimulating, acts positively on lethargy and tiredness. Useful in meditation. • Blends well with cardamom, lavendin, rosemary, and rosewood.	Topical, room diffusion, massage	• Mediterranean, India • Steam • Seeds and fruit • Middle to Top	Photosensitizing.
Cypress (*cupressus sempervirens*)	• Refreshing, sweet-balsamic scent. • Balancing, warming, uplifting, and energizing. Antiseptic, astringent, and circulatory stimulant. Useful for bronchial complaints and is a choice spasmolytic for whooping cough. Decongestant for prostate, veins, and the lymphatic system. Strengthens a weak pancreas. Helps prevent the spread of varicose veins, hemorrhoids, and edema, especially of the lower limbs. Regulates female hormonal systems. • Blends well with juniper, lavender, pine, and sandalwood.	Topical, bath, room diffusion, inhalation massage	• Southern Europe, France, Asia, Germany, Italy • Steam • Leaves and fruits • Middle to Base	Avoid in women with breast cancer. Avoid in glaucoma. Use with caution in pregnancy.
Dill (*anethum graveolens*)	• Light, fresh, warm, spicy aroma. • Improves digestion, soothes intestines, relieves flatulence. Calming and relaxing. Relieves pain and menstrual discomfort. Calms headaches and helps with excess sweating due to nervous tension. It can stimulate milk flow in nursing mothers. • Blends well with caraway, citruses, elemi, and nutmeg.	Topical, bath, room diffusion, inhalation, massage	• Mediterranean, Russia • Steam • Seeds and whole plant • Middle	

Essential Oil Common Name (*botanical name*)	Aroma Traditional and/or documented uses Blending	Methods of Use	Country of Origin Distillation Method Part of the Plant Note	Precautions
Elemi (*canarium luzonicum*)	• Light, fresh, balsamic, spicy scent. • Warming, improves circulation. Calming, relaxing, reduces stress, promotes a restful sleep. Opens the breathing passages for deeper breathing, mildly breaks up mucous. Mood uplifting, helps one to communicate with inner feelings. Heals skin tissue. Helpful for meditation. • Blends well with frankincense, lavender, myrrh, sage, and spices.	Topical, bath, inhalation, massage	• Asia • Steam • Wood • Middle	
Eucalyptus, Narrow-leaved Peppermint (*e. radiata*)	• Refreshing and medicinal. • Antibacterial, antiviral, expectorant. Useful in respiratory and anti-inflammatory treatments and for rhinitis, flu, otitis, sinusitis, bronchitis, and cough. Good for children. • Blends well with benzoin, citruses, lavender, and other tree oils.	Topical, bath, room diffusion, inhalation, massage	• Australia, Tasmania • Steam • Leaves and twigs • Top	
Eucalyptus, Lemon (*e. citriodora*)	• Fresh, lemon scent. • Used as antibiotic by early settlers and possibly Aboriginals as astringent for the treatment of diarrhea. Anti-inflammatory and analgesic for arthritis. Relieves muscular tensions, muscle cramps, sprains, sore tendons, and carpal tunnel injuries. Sedative, uplifting, and reviving, helpful in fatigue. Antiseptic, useful for respiratory and skin conditions. • Blends well with benzoin, citruses, lavender, and other tree oils.	Topical, room diffusion, inhalation, massage	• Australia, Tasmania • Steam • Leaves and twigs • Top	Potential skin irritant. Use with caution in pregnancy.

Eucalyptus, Broad-leaved Peppermint (*e. dives*)	• Camphorous, spicy, and mint scented. • Mucolytic for bronchitis. Antiseptic, expectorant, anti-inflammatory, antifungal, insectifugal. Used for oily and congested skin. • Blends well with citruses, mint oils, and other tree oils.	Topical, bath, room diffusion, inhalation, massage	• Australia, Tasmania • Steam • Leaves • Top	Contains ketones; Avoid in children less than 10 years old and in pregnancy.
Eucalyptus, Blue Gum (*e. globulus*)	• Strong, camphorous scent. • Expectorant and antiseptic; suitable for cold symptoms, bronchitis, catarrh, flu, and sinusitis. A respiratory anti-inflammatory useful in asthma. Stimulating and cooling, it is used in inhalations for deep bronchial infection or in massage oil for muscular aches, sluggish circulation, and arthritic complaints. • Blends well with citruses, mint oils, and other tree oils.	Topical, bath, room diffusion, inhalation, massage	• Australia, Tasmania • Steam • Leaves and twigs • Top	Not to be used with small children because of high cineole content. Use with caution in pregnancy.
Eucalyptus, Blue Mallee (*e. Polybractea, cryptone type*)	• Less camphorous odor than Blue Gum variety. • Expectorant, good relief for head colds. Used for condylomas, uterine, and genital warts, and viral dysplasia. Prostate decongestant. Antiparasitic and antimalarial. Helpful for rheumatism and muscular pain. • Blends well with citruses, lavender, and other tree oils.	Topical, bath, room diffusion, inhalation, massage	• Australia, Tasmania • Steam • Leaves • Top	Especially suited for improving room air with a diffuser. Use with caution in pregnancy.
Eucalyptus (*e. smithii*)	• Strong, camphorous, clean scent. • Anti-infective and antiviral; its expectorant properties help with bronchitis and catarrh. The oil is commonly used in steam inhalation for colds and flu. It can also be used as a vapor bath and inhaled for asthma and other respiratory ailments, and is an antiseptic bath addition. An effective chest rub. A digestive stimulant. • Blends well with citruses and other tree oils.	Topical, bath, room diffusion, inhalation, massage	• Australia, Tasmania • Steam • Leaves • Top	

Essential Oil Common Name (*botanical name*)	Aroma Traditional and/or documented uses Blending	Methods of Use	Country of Origin Distillation Method Part of the Plant Note	Precautions
Eucalyptus (*e. staigeriana*)	• Wonderful lemony, clean scent. • Anti-infective, antiviral, antiseptic, expectorant, and anti-inflammatory, digestive stimulant, decongestant. Used in perfumery and flavoring. • Blends well with citruses, lavender, and other tree oils.	Topical, bath, room diffusion, inhalation, massage	• Australia, Tasmania • Steam • Leaves • Top	
Everlasting, Helichrysum (*helichrysum italicum*)	• Warm, pungent, herbal aroma. • Anti-inflammatory, antihemotoma, and skin-regenerating activity. Excellent for scars. Good mucolytic, useful for coughs. Effective for joint pain associated with rheumatoid arthritis. • Blends well with chamomile, eucalyptus citriodora, lavender, rosemary, and yarrow.	Topical, bath, massage, inhalation	• Mediterranean, Asia, Europe • Steam • Flowers • Middle	Not to be used during pregnancy due to its anticoagulant effects.
Fennel (*foeniculum vulgare*)	• Spicy, warm, and sweet, similar to anise. • Stimulates estrogen; useful for ovarian problems, PMS, and menopause. In a diffuser, fennel can be used to stimulant the appetite. Carminative; useful for a bloated abdomen, colic, constipation, other digestive problems. Used in a base cream or lotion, fennel oil can be helpful for general skin care and especially for bruises, dull, oily and mature skins. Helpful for cellulite, rheumatism, and edema. • Blends well with aniseed, black pepper, coriander, and cumin.	Topical, bath, room diffusion, inhalation, massage	• California, India, Japan, Central Europe, England, Mediterranean • Steam • Crushed seeds • Top to Middle	Best avoided in pregnancy until the last 2 months. Avoid in babies and children. Not to be used by women with breast cancer. Avoid in epilepsy, and kidney problems.

Fir, Silver (*abies alba*) Fir (*albies siberica*)	• Sweet, rich scent. • Palliative for rheumatic muscle aches and pains. Reduces coughing from lung congestion, bronchitis, or asthma. Stimulating, increases energy. Considered useful for its grounding effects. Warming and beneficial in massage blends to relieve muscular aches and pains. • Blends well with citruses, cedarwood, frankincense, lavender, and rosemary.	Topical, bath, inhalation, massage	• North America, Europe • Steam • Needles • Middle	Use in asthma as a preventative, rather than for acute attack. Use with caution in pregnancy.
Fir, Douglas (*pseudotsuga menziesii*)	• Fresh, green, powerful, and clean. • Powerful and elevating. Refreshing, reviving, improves mental clarity. Purifying, a respiratory and breath cleanser. Opens sinuses and breathing passages. Removes lymphatic deposits and helps in cellulite reduction. Encourages communication. • Blends well with cedarwood, citruses, frankincense, and lavender.	Topical, bath, inhalation, massage	• North America, Europe • Steam • Needles • Middle	Use with caution in pregnancy.
Frankincense (Olibanum) (*boswellia carterii*)	• Sweet, rich, and woody. • Useful for asthma, bronchitis, and weakened immune system. Helps with catarrh symptoms. Calms anxiety and balances mood swings; good for mental fatigue, depression, and pain relief. Helpful for skin regeneration, anti aging wrinkle prevention, mature and dry skin, and to calm inflammatory processes. Traditionally used for ceremonial incense, meditation, and perfumery. • Blends well with citruses, myrrh, sandalwood, and spices.	Topical, bath, room diffusion, massage, perfume	• East Africa, China, Southern Arabia, Iran, Lebanon • Steam, CO_2 • Resin from bark • Base	

Essential Oil Common Name (*botanical name*)	Aroma Traditional and/or documented uses Blending	Methods of Use	Country of Origin Distillation Method Part of the Plant Note	Precautions
Galbanum (*ferula galbaniflua*)	• Green, balsamic, and woody aroma. • Used for respiratory ailments. Calming, reduces stress. Anti-inflammatory; used to relieve poor circulation and muscular aches and pains. Excellent for mature or wrinkled skin, acne, abscesses, cuts. Effective in healing scar tissue. Aphrodisiac. • Blends well with elemi, fir, frankincense, geranium, ginger, jasmine, lavender, and palmarosa.	Topical, bath, inhalation, massage	• Iran, Lebanon, Mediterranean • Steam • Resin from bark • Middle to Base	
Geranium (*pelargonium graviolens*)	• Rose-like, green, and flowery. • Uplifting, balancing, soothing, and relaxing. Useful in female issues. Antidepressant. Antifungal, especially against candida albicans, without affecting the bacterial flora. Stops bleeding, helpful to bruises. Stimulates the functions of the liver and pancreas. Excellent for all skin types. • Blends well with bergamot, citruses, lavender, neroli, and rose.	Topical, bath, room diffusion, inhalation, massage, perfume	• Algeria, Egypt, Madagascar, China, Guinea, France, Morocco, Russia • Steam • Whole plant • Middle to Top	Use with caution in pregnancy.
Ginger (*zingiber officinale*)	• Sharp, spicy, warming, and strengthening. • Antispasmodic, benefits digestive problems, and is immune-strengthening. Reduces inflammation and relieves pain (especially in rheumatic disorders and migraine headaches) by inhibiting cyclooxygenase and lipoxygenase enzyme activity. Protects against gastric mucosal lesions. Useful for fatigue and nervous exhaustion. Aphrodisiac and sexual tonic. • Blends well with cedarwood, citruses, frankincense, and resins.	Topical, room diffusion, inhalation, massage, perfumery	• India, West Indies, Africa, China, Japan, Philippines, Tahiti • Root • Steam • Middle to Base	Avoid use on sensitive or damaged skin.

Goldenrod (*solidago canadensis*)	• Fresh, crisp, and herbaceous. • Warming, relaxing, and calming. Supports the circulatory system, urinary tract, and liver function. Historically, a valuable remedy for urinary tract disorders. It is used both for serious ailments such as nephritis and for more common problems like cystitis. Goldenrod's saponins act specifically against the Candida fungus. Can also be used for sore throats and chronic nasal congestion. It may be used as a mouthwash or douche for yeast infections. • Blends well with citruses and wood oils.	Topical, room diffusion, inhalation, massage	• Canada • Steam • Flowering herb • Middle to top	damaged skin. Avoid in pregnancy, with babies & children.
Grapefruit (*citrus paradisi*)	• Light, sweet, and refreshing. Pink grapefruit is a little sweeter than white grapefruit oil. • Uplifting, stimulating, and reviving. Stabilizes manic-depression. A lymphatic stimulant, detoxyifing; has an effect on obesity, cellulite, and water retention. Has a cleansing effect on the kidneys and vascular system. Liver tonic. Antiseptic. Specific as a tonic for oily or congested skin. • Blends well with bergamot, citruses, cypress, geranium, lavender, and palmarosa.	Topical, bath, room diffusion, inhalation, massage	• US, Israel • Expressed • Peel • Top	Photosensitizing.
Guaiacwood (*bulnesia sarmienti*)	• Sweet, smoky, and earthy-rose aroma. • Calming, relaxing, reduces stress/tension, enhances a restful sleep. Mood uplifter, improves mental clarity, helpful in meditation. Purifying to the tissues. Useful for rheumatoid arthritis, chronic rheumatism, and gout, relieving pain and inflammation. It is a mild laxative and diuretic. • Blends well with amyris, bergamot, elemi, frankincense, geranium, grapefruit, jasmine, lavender, neroli, oakmoss, palmarosa, patchouli, rose, sandalwood, and ylang ylang.	Topical, room diffusion, bath, inhalation, massage, perfumery	• Paraguay • Steam • Heart Wood and sawdust • Base	

Essential Oil Common Name (*botanical name*)	**Aroma Traditional and/or documented uses Blending**	**Methods of Use**	**Country of Origin Distillation Method Part of the Plant Note**	**Precautions**
Helichrysum Rambiazina (*helichrysum gymnocephalum*)	• Sweet, fruity, and rich. • Cooling, opens breathing, encourages deeper breathing, and promotes alertness. Useful for the treatment of rheumatism, herpes, hematoma, varicose ulcers, dermatitis, and gingivitis. • Blends well with citruses, clary sage, geranium, lavender, rose, lavender, and spice oils.	Topical, bath, massage, inhalation	• Madagascar • Steam • Whole plant • Middle	
Hyssop (*hyssop offiinalis ssp. decumbens*)	• Warm, spicy, and camphorous. • Sympathotonic. Calming and refreshing, useful for all nervous depression. Antiviral; helpful in upper respiratory conditions and asthma-related lung inflammation. Facilitates metabolic and liver secretions. • Blends well with bay, citruses, clary sage, geranium, lavender, myrtle, and rosemary	Topical, room diffusion, massage, inhalation	• Europe, Asia, Brazil • Steam • Flowering tops and leaves • Middle	*Hyssop officinalis*: contains high ketone content--avoid use in epilepsy and glaucoma. Avoid in pregnancy and hypertension.
Jade Cypress (*callitris glaucophylla*)	• Warm and woodsy with green and earthy undertones. • Traditionally used for colds and sores. Good fixative or to add an earthy note to a perfume blend. • Blends well with citruses, florals, green scents, lavender, and lemon myrtle.	Topical, bath, massage, inhalation, perfume	• Australia • Steam • Leaves and twigs • Base	

Jasmine (*jasmimum grandiflorum*) (*jasmimum sambac*)	• Intensely floral and heavy. • Facilitates delivery in childbirth; it hastens the birth by strengthening the contractions and at the same time relieving the pain. A hormone balancer, relieves spasm in the uterus. Aphrodisiac. Remedy for severe depression, nervous tension, stress, and insomnia. It soothes the nerves and produces a feeling of confidence, optimism, and euphoria. It revitalizes and restores energy. Tones dry, oily, irritated, and sensitive skin. Often used to assist with stretch marks and scarring. • Blends well with most citrus, floral, and wood oils.	Topical, bath, massage, perfume	• Algeria, Morocco, France, China, Egypt, Italy, Turkey. • Enfleurage, solvent extraction, CO2 • Flowers • Base	Caution in pregnancy (okay after 16 weeks).
Juniper (*juniperus communis*)	• Refreshing, woody-sweet scent. • Digestive tonic effective for cirrhosis. A diuretic and pancreatic stimulant. Has a general augmenting action on mucous secretions. Aids active elimination of unwanted materials in the joints, and is helpful for gout and arthritis. Cleansing tonic for oily skin and acne. Uplifting and stimulating, aids in mental exhaustion. • Blends well with bergamot, cypress, frankincense, lavender, rosemary, and sandalwood.	Topical, bath, room diffusion, inhalation, massage	• Canada, France, Italy, Morocco, North Asia, Spain, Sweden • Steam • Berries • Middle	Not to be used where there is inflammation of the kidneys. Use with caution in pregnancy.
Kanuka (*kunzea ericoides*)	• Sweet, herbaceous, earthy, similar to the aroma of Manuka. • Antibiotic, disinfectant. Useful in acne preparations, foot care, oral hygiene products, skin and hair care. Anti-inflammatory; relieves muscular pain and swelling due to sprains, strains, and sports injuries. Promotes calmness. • Blends well with citruses, lavender, other wood oils.	Topical, bath, room diffusion, inhalation, massage	• New Zealand • Steam • Leaves and Small stems • Middle	

Essential Oil Common Name (*botanical name*)	Aroma Traditional and/or documented uses Blending	Methods of Use	Country of Origin Distillation Method Part of the Plant Note	Precautions
Katafray (*cedrelopsis grevei*)	• Sharp, fresh, herbaceous, and green. • Relaxing and reduces stress. Fortifying and tonic, traditionally used by woman after giving birth. This plant is one of the most commonly used in Madagascar especially to relieve rheumatic pains. • Blends well with citrus and wood oils.	Topical, bath, room diffusion, inhalation, massage	• Madagascar • Steam • Bark of the tree • Middle	
Kunzea (*kunzea ambigua*)	• Clean balsamic scent with fresh invigorating undertones. • Antiseptic, antifungal; effective against staph, candida, and pseudomonas. Helpful in eczema, dermatitis, nail infections, and leg ulcers. Useful for arthritic relief, muscular aches and pains, nervous tension, stress, and symptoms of influenza. • Blends well with citruses, lavender, lemon myrtle, peppermint, and rosalina.	Topical, bath, room diffusion, inhalation, massage	• Australia, Tasmania • Steam • Leaves • Middle	
Labdanum (Rockrose) (*cistus ladaniferus*)	• Warm, sweet, herbaceous, and musky scent. • Increases circulation. A good choice as an addition to a lymph drainage massage blend. Calming, reduces stress, mood uplifting, euphoric, and centering. Brings out feelings, encourages communication. Helpful for meditation. Used for treating mature skin, dry skin, and wrinkles. Used as a fixative. • Blends well with bergamot, chamomile, citruses, clary sage, frankincense, juniper, lavender, patchouli, pine, sandalwood, and vetiver.	Topical, inhalation, massage, perfume	• Mediterranean, Middle East • Steam • Resin from leaves • Middle to Base	

Lantana (*lantana camara*)	• Herbaceous and spicy. • Strong mucolytic, useful for chronic bronchitis and asthma. Treats varicose ulcers. Cooling, calming, reduces stress. Supports a deep sleep. Mood uplifting. • Blends well with citrus and wood oils.	Topical, bath, inhalation, massage	• US • Steam • Leaves • Middle	Neurotoxic and abortive. Use small amounts.
Lavender (*lavendula angustifolia*) (*lavendula officinalis*) (*lavendula vera*)	• Floral, sweet, herbal scent. • Considered one of the most universally useful oils. Balancing, calming, relaxing, soothing; relieves tension and pain. Promotes deep restful sleep. Analgesic, hypotensive, and cicatrizant. A must for every first aid kit, it can be used to relieve insect bits and healing small cuts, and is useful for burns, sunburns, stings, muscular aches, cuts, blemishes, bruises, headaches, insect bites, colds, flu, stress, and menstrual cramps. It is excellent for all skin types. May be applied neat (undiluted) to the skin. • Blends well with other citruses, flower oils, marjoram, and rosemary.	Topical, bath, room diffusion, inhalation, massage, perfume	• France, Spain, England, Bulgaria, Tasmania • Steam • Flowers • Middle	
Lavender, Spike (*lavendula latifolia*)	• Fresh, camphorous, and woody aroma. • Effective for bronchitis and laryngitis as an expectorant and antiviral. Analgesic; lessens muscular and rheumatic pain promoting relaxation of the nerve fibers. Antidepressant. • Blends well with citruses, clary sage, cypress, geranium, pine, and rosemary.	Topical, bath, room diffusion, inhalation, massage	• France, Spain, England • Steam • Flowers • Middle	Small children and pregnant women should use only with extreme caution.

Essential Oil Common Name (*botanical name*)	**Aroma Traditional and/or documented uses Blending**	**Methods of Use**	**Country of Origin Distillation Method Part of the Plant Note**	**Precautions**
Lavendin (*lavendula intermedia*)	• Fresh, camphorous, and flowery aroma. • Antiviral, antifungal, neurotonic. Antidepressant. Analgesic, useful for aches, pains, and muscle stiffness. • Blends well with bay, cinnamon, citruses, clary sage, clove, cypress, geranium, pine, and rosemary.	Topical, bath, room diffusion, inhalation, massage	• France, Spain, England • Steam • Flowers • Middle	
Lemon (*citrus limon*)	• Clean, light, sharp, and fresh. • Anti-infectious, antiviral, antibacterial. Useful in blends aimed at liver regeneration and detoxification. Stimulates digestion. Useful for gallstones and urinary stones; a pancreatic stimulant. Uplifting, refreshing. Cleansing and astringent treatment for oily skin. • Blends well with other citruses, geranium, lavender, and neroli.	Topical, bath, room diffusion, inhalation, massage	• Brazil, Spain, US, Israel • Expressed • Peel of the green fruit • Top	Photosensitizing.
Lemongrass (*cymbopogen citratus*)	• Pungent and lemony. • Anti-inflammatory; contracts weak connective tissues and tones the skin. Sedative. Balances the autonomic nervous system and acts as a vasodilator. Improves digestion. Improves alertness. Uplifting. Astringent, antibacterial, antiviral. A diuretic, useful for cellulite. Stimulating hair treatment. Good room deodorizer. • Blends well with clary sage, geranium, jasmine, and lavender.	Topical, bath, inhalation, massage, room diffusion	• Asia, Central Africa • Steam • Whole plant • Top	Skin irritant if not well blended. Photosensitizing. Avoid in pregnancy.

Lemon Myrtle (*backhousia citriadora*)	• Clean, sharp, sweet, lemon scent. • Antiseptic, antiviral, antibacterial; helpful in respiratory conditions to open sinus passages. Supports and strengthens the immune system. Effective against staph, clostridium, aspergillus, and candida. Uplifting and refreshing, useful for concentration and clearing the mind. An anti-stress oil, provides relaxation and mental rejuvenation. Reduces pain and discomfort. • Blends well with other wood and citrus oils, lavender, vetiver, other wood oils, and ylang ylang.	Topical, bath, room diffusion, inhalation, massage	• Australia • Steam • Leaf • Middle	
Lemon Scented Tea Tree (*leptospermum petersonii*)	• Pleasant, sharp, lemony floral scent. • Anti-infective, antiviral, antiseptic, expectorant. Digestive stimulant. Anti-inflammatory; relieves aches and pains and looses tight muscles. Calming, reduces stress and tension. Useful for treatment of oily skin and acne. • Blends well with cypress, rosewood, and sandalwood.	Topical, bath, inhalation, massage	• New Zealand, Australia • Steam • Leaves and branches • Middle	
Lemon verbena (*lippia citriodora*)	• Lemony, sweet, and fresh. • Calming, antidepressant. Relieves anxiety, insomnia, and nervous tension. Reviving, improves mental clarity and alertness. Works on the psycho-hormonal level. Anti-inflammatory. Calms heart palpitations and may deal with nervous insomnia. A cooling action on the liver mitigates inflammation and infection, as in cirrhosis. • Blends well with citruses, elemi, neroli, and palmarosa.	Topical, inhalation, massage	• South America • Steam • Leaves and branches • Middle to Top	Photosensitizing. Use with caution in pregnancy.

Essential Oil Common Name (*botanical name*)	**Aroma Traditional and/or documented uses Blending**	**Methods of Use**	**Country of Origin Distillation Method Part of the Plant Note**	**Precautions**
Lime (*citrus aurantifolia*) (*citrus latifolia*)	• Refreshing, tart, cooling, and uplifting. • A tonic to the immune system, and is useful to cool fevers associated with colds, sore throats, and the flu. Helps reduce cellulite. Useful for rheumatic pain. Stimulates digestive secretions, and encourages appetite. Astringent and toning action to clear oily skin and acne. Refreshes a tired mind and helps with depression. • Blends well with florals, spice and wood oils.	Topical, bath, room diffusion, inhalation, massage	• Asia, Mexico, US, Brazil, Italy • Expressed • Peel • Top	Photosensitizing.
Lovage (*levisticum officinalis*)	• Celery-like, rich, spicy warm, and fresh. • Minimal usage for digestive complaints. • Blends well with bay, galbanum, lavendin, opopanax, rose, and spice oils.	Perfumery	• UK, France • Steam • Leaves • Top to middle	Avoid during pregnancy.
Mandarin (*citrus reticulata*)	• Light, sweet, floral scent. • Antispasmodic for cardiovascular, digestive, and respiratory systems. Calms activity of sympathetic nervous system and soothes restlessness, especially hyperactive children. Stimulates liver, helping to regulate metabolic process and aids in the secretion of bile and breakdown of fats. • Blends well with other citruses and spice oils.	Topical, bath, room diffusion, inhalation, massage	• Asia, US, Brazil, Argentina, China • Expressed • Peel • Top	Photosensitizing.

Manuka (*leptospermum scoparium*)	• Woody, earthy, and balsamic. • Antibacterial, anti-acne, antihistamine, antiallergenic. Antifungal; useful for athlete's foot, skin infections, ringworm, thrush, and nail bed infections. Anti-inflammatory, relaxes tired and aching muscles and joints. Beneficial for stress, nervousness, and anxiety that manifest as rashes, itching, and nasal problems. • Blends well with citruses and lavender.	Topical, bath, room diffusion, inhalation, massage	• New Zealand • Steam • Leaf and seed capsule • Middle	
Marjoram, Sweet (*origanum marjorana*)	• Woody, herbal aroma. • Antibacterial with spasmolytic properties; useful for colds and congestion. Analgesic, effective for arthritis, muscular pain, and rheumatism. A neurotonic; balances the parasympathetic nervous system. Sedative; good for tension and anxiety. Anaphrodisiac. • Blends well with bergamot, eucalyptus, lavender, orange, rosemary, and ylang ylang.	Topical, bath, room diffusion, inhalation, massage	• France, England, Mediterranean, Egypt, Spain, Hungary • Steam • Flowering Tops • Middle	
Massoia Bark (*cryptocaria massoia*)	• Rich, slightly floral scent. • Warming, improves circulation. Calming, relaxing, mood uplifting, aphrodisiac, euphoric, reviving, and heightens the senses. • Blends well with benzoin, vanilla, lavender, rose, ylang ylang, and orange.	Topical, room diffusion, inhalation, massage, perfume	• Indonesia, New Guinea • Steam • Tree bark • Base	Skin irritant and should be used with caution.

Essential Oil Common Name (*botanical name*)	Aroma Traditional and/or documented uses Blending	Methods of Use	Country of Origin Distillation Method Part of the Plant Note	Precautions
May Chang (*litsea cubeba*)	• Intense, lemony, fresh aroma. • Anti-inflammatory, calming, sedative. Useful in "low energy" states, improves mental clarity and alertness, anxiety, and depression. Tonic for heart and respiratory system; a bronchodilator. Digestive stimulant, improves the appetite, and helps indigestion. Assists with tissue toning and cellulite reduction. • Blends well with wood oils.	Topical, room diffusion, inhalation, massage	• Europe • Steam • Fruit • Top	Skin irritant if not well blended. Avoid with glaucoma. May have a hormone-like action. Avoid in prostatic hyperplasia.
Melissa (Lemon Balm) (*melissa officinalis*)	• Tart lemon and herbal scent. • Soothing, uplifting, and calming; relieves depression, stress, and insomnia. Powerful sedative; ameliorates anger in crisis or trauma. Calming in times of emotional shock and grief. Antiviral, effective for herpes lesions and candida. Anti-inflammatory when highly diluted. Useful in headaches, vertigo, morning sickness, and hypertension. • Blends well with citruses, florals, geranium, lavender, and rose.	Topical, room diffusion, inhalation, massage	• Europe, Mediterranean • Steam • Leaves • Top to Middle	Useful in low concentrations (i.e. 1: 100)
Myrrh (*commiphora myrrhal*)	• Heavy, rich, thick, and resinous. • Powerful anti-inflammatory, antiviral, astringent, and gentle expectorant; useful for coughs, colds, and bronchitis. Deflates sexual over excitation. Binds to opioid receptors for its analgesic effects. Helps regulate an overactive thyroid. Good for mature skin, dry scalp, chapped skin, and open wounds. Fixative for perfume. • Blends well with frankincense, geranium, juniper, lavender, mandarin, mints, and spice	Topical, bath, room inhalation, massage, perfume	• Africa, Asia • Steam, CO2 • Resin from bark • Base	Avoid in pregnancy.

Myrtle (*myrtus communis*)	• Sweet, fresh, floral, and camphorous. Expectorant; combats excess moisture, bronchial catarrh, and clears sinusitis. Useful for hay fever and pulmonary disorders. Regenerating to the skin. Promotes restful sleep. Good for acne, oily skin, and open pores. • Blends well with clary sage, ginger, and lavender.	Topical, bath, room diffusion, inhalation, massage	• Europe, Asia • Steam • Leaves, twigs and flowering tops • Top to Middle	Use with caution in pregnancy.
Neroli (*citrus bigaradia, aurantium*) "flowers"	• Floral, warm, and soothing. • Strengthening. Useful for anxiety, nervous depression, insomnia, PMS, and shock. Facilitates birthing and eases postpartum depression. A hepatic and pancreatic stimulant. Tonifying for most skin types, but especially mature skin lacking vitality and suppleness. Can help with the regenerating of skin cells and is useful for scar tissue and stretch marks. • Blends well with bergamot, orange, petitgrain, and rose.	Topical, bath, inhalation, massage, perfume	• India, China, Tunisia, France, Italy, California, South America, West Indies • Enfleurage, steam, or solvent extraction • Blossoms • Middle to Base	
Nerolina (*melaleuca quinquenervia)*	• Soft, sweet, fruity, "green" aroma. • Antiseptic, antispasmodic, bactericidal, and a skin toner. Soothes respiratory tract. Calming, soothing, and uplifting. Useful for fatigue, stress, and adrenal exhaustion. • Blends well with citrus and floral oils.	Topical, bath, room diffusion, massage	• Australia • Steam • Leaves and small stems • Middle	

Essential Oil Common Name (*botanical name*)	Aroma Traditional and/or documented uses Blending	Methods of Use	Country of Origin Distillation Method Part of the Plant Note	Precautions
Niaouli (*melaleuca quinquenervia viridiflora*)	• Sweet herbal, earthy, menthol scent. • Stimulates the defense mechanisms of the body. Broadly antiseptic, antiviral, antifungal, and antiparasitic; an expectorant. Effective for asthma, sinusitis, bronchitis, and viral hepatitis. Endocrine tonic with special affinity to pituitary and ovarian glands. Good for hemorrhoids, herpes, and varicose veins. Estrogen-like characteristics. Good skin toner. • Blends well with eucalyptus, fir, and rosemary.	Topical, bath, room diffusion, inhalation, massage	• Australia, Tasmania, East Indies • Steam • Leaves and small stems • Middle	Should be used with caution in children less than 10 years, and in pregnancy.
Nutmeg (*myristica fragrans*)	• Sensual, warm, and spicy. • Analgesic, antibacterial, carminative, digestive stimulant. Emmenagogic, reproductive tonic, uterotonic. Imitates estrogen, aids in birthing by strengthening contractions. Warming quality to muscular aches and pains. Invigorating to the heart and circulation. • Blends well with florals, spices, and wood oils.	Topical, bath, room diffusion, inhalation, massage	• Sri Lanka, West Indies, Java, Sumatra, Indonesia • Steam • Seeds • Middle	Avoid in pregnancy. Can cause stupefying effects.
Oakmoss (*evernia prunasti*)	• Earthy, mossy, and green scent. • Uplifting, cooling, and calming, it is reputed as an aphrodisiac. Fixative in perfumes. Antiseptic. Properties are more emotional and spiritual than physical. • Blends well with cedarwood, citruses, florals, pine, and vetiver.	Perfume, blended for massage or inhalation, perfumery	• Europe, North America, Algeria • Solvent extraction • Resin • Base	

Opoponax (*commiphoria erythraea*)	• Sweet, woody, root-like scent. Similar to myrrh. • Antiseptic, antispasmodic, expectorant. It is used to guard against negative influences, strengthen the senses, and to increase awareness and intuition. Used as a fixative in perfume. • Blends well with bergamot, clary sage, frankincense, fir, labdanum, myrrh, patchouli, sandalwood, and vetiver.	Topical, room diffusion, inhalation, massage, perfumery	• Kenya, Somalia • Steam or Solvent extraction • Resin • Middle to Base	
Orange, Sweet (*citrus simensis*) Orange, Blood (*citrus simensis var sanguina*)	• Sweet and citrus. Blood orange is richer and sweeter. • Calming and relaxing, especially for angry and irritable children. Useful for anxiety, insomnia, and nervousness. Antispasmodic. Stimulates bile and could help digestion of fats and eliminate toxins. Good for oily skin. • Blends well with frankincense, lavender, and spice oils.	Topical, bath, room diffusion, inhalation, massage	• US, Israel, Brazil, France, Spain • Fruit peel • Expressed • Top	Photosensitizing.
Oregano (*origanum compactum*) (*origanum vulgare*)	• Spicy-herbaceous and warm. • Antibacterial, antifungal, antiparasitic. Useful in respiratory conditions. Strong antioxidant and anti-inflammatory effects, useful for CFS and/or fibromyalgia. Soothes the stomach, liver, and spleen. Warming, it improves circulation. • Blends well with lavendin, oakmoss, pine, rosemary, and cedarwood.	Topical, room diffusion, inhalation, massage	• Europe, North Africa, Egypt, Asia, US • Steam • Flowers • Middle	Not for asthmatics. Skin irritant, best used highly diluted. Use with caution in pregnancy. Avoid in children.

Essential Oil Common Name (*botanical name*)	**Aroma Traditional and/or documented uses Blending**	**Methods of Use**	**Country of Origin Distillation Method Part of the Plant Note**	**Precautions**
Palmarosa (*cymbopogon martinii*)	• Rosy-floral, sweet, green, and soothing. • Antiviral, antibacterial, antifungal. Useful in rhinitis, sinusitis, bronchitis, intestinal flu, cystitis, vaginitis, acne, and eczema. A uterine, neuro- and cardio tonic. Balancing and regenerative for dry, mature, cracked, or chapped skin. Stimulating; useful in stress, exhaustion, and nervousness. • Blends well with cedarwood, coriander, florals, geranium, petitgrain, and wood oils.	Topical, bath, room diffusion, inhalation, massage	• Asia, Brazil, Central America • Steam • Whole plant (grass) • Middle to Top	
Parsley (*petroselium sativum*)	• Strong, spicy-herbaceous aroma. • Stimulates the kidneys and is a strong diuretic; helpful in menstrual water retention, edema, and cellulite. Cleansing action on blood, tonic effect on circulation, helps ease rheumatism and arthritis. Tonic to the liver. Antispasmodic specific to colon and nervous system. Imitates estrogen. • Blends well with clary sage, spice oils, and tea tree.	Topical, inhalation, massage	• Mediterranean, Europe, Africa • Steam • Seeds • Middle	Avoid in pregnancy, kidney disease and peptic ulcers. Photosensitizing.

Patchouli (*pogostemon cablin*)	• Earthy and sweet. • Anti-inflammatory; useful in acne, hemorrhoids, and varicose veins. A tissue regenerator; helps regrowth of skin cells and formation of scar tissue. Specific for mature, oily, cracked, or chapped skin, and oily hair. Warming, calming, and grounding. Stimulating; aphrodisiac and euphoric. Antiseptic and antifungal. • Blends well with citruses, jasmine, neroli, rose, and wood oils.	Topical, bath, inhalation, massage	• Asia, Madagascar, Japan • Steam • Leaves • Base	
Pennyroyal (*mentha pulegium*)	• Pleasant, fresh aroma. • Oil used externally to wards off fleas, ants, gnats, lice, mosquitoes, ticks, and moths. • Blends with citronella, geranium, lavendin, rosemary, and sage.	Topical, diluted in a spray	• England • Steam • Leaves • Top	Toxic and an abortifacient and can even in small quantities cause acute liver and lung damage.
Peppermint (*mentha x piperita*)	• Sharp, minty, stimulating, and refreshing. • Instant relief from nausea, travel sickness, and indigestion. Most effective essential oil for stimulating liver. Cooling and anti-inflammatory. Can open congested sinuses. Analgesic, especially for headaches...Apply a 15% dilution to forehead, neck, shoulders. Stimulating; useful for exhaustion and fatigue. • Blends well with benzoin, eucalyptus, lavender, lemon, other mints, and rosemary.	Topical, room diffusion, inhalation, massage	• US, Japan, Great Britain, Brazil, China, France • Steam • Leaves and flowering tips • Top	Not for children under 2 and a half years. Avoid in insomnia. Use with caution in pregnancy.

Essential Oil Common Name (*botanical name*)	Aroma Traditional and/or documented uses Blending	Methods of Use	Country of Origin Distillation Method Part of the Plant Note	Precautions
Petitgrain (*citrus aurantium var. amara*) "leaves"	• Fresh citrus-floral, and "green." • Antispasmodic, sedative, anxiolytic. Calms the high-strung; useful in stress and anxiety. Clarifying and uplifting in mental fatigue. Eases breathing and relaxes muscle spasms. A skin tonic. Used extensively in perfumery. • Blends well with balsams, bergamot, clary sage, clove, geranium, labdanum, lavender, oakmoss, and rosemary.	Topical, bath, room diffusion, inhalation, massage, perfume	• Asia, India, France, Italy, Brazil, Paraguay • Steam • Leaves, twigs, and unripe green fruit • Top	
Pine, Longleaf (*pinus palustris*)	• Sweet, balsamic, pinewood scent. • Mild analgesic, antiseptic, bactericidal, expectorant. Useful for muscular aches and pains and stiffness. Helpful in bronchitis, catarrh, and sinusitis. • Blends well with cedarwood, lemon, oakmoss, and rosemary.	Topical, bath, room diffusion, inhalation, massage	• US • Steam • Sawdust and wood chips • Middle	Use with caution in pregnancy. Possibly irritating to sensitive skin.
Pine, Scotch (*pinus sylvestris*) Pine, Ocean (Sea) (*pinus pinaster*)	• Fresh, stimulating evergreen aroma. • Anti-infectious, antifungal. Upper respiratory tract decongestant; useful for colds, coughs, sinus infections, and asthma. Tonic and adrenal stimulant, promotes vitality. Good for hypotension. Neurotonic. Useful for muscle and joint pain. Refreshing and reviving, improves alertness, and memory. • Blends well with cedarwood, eucalyptus, lavender, lemon, marjoram, niaouli, sage, and tea tree.	Topical, bath, room diffusion, inhalation, massage	• Asia, Europe, US • Steam • Needles and small branches • Middle	10% topically over kidney area for adrenal support. Has a strong diuretic effect. Avoid in insomnia. Use with caution in pregnancy. Possibly irritating to sensitive skin.

Ravensara (*ravensara aromatica*)	• Camphorous, pungent scent. • Antiseptic and antiviral. Expectorant; helps with flu, sinusitis, bronchitis. Choice in acute influenza and shingles. Nerve tonic, raises overall energy and creates an optimistic mood. Calming, useful for insomnia; a muscle relaxant. • Blends well with benzoin, citruses, rosemary, and tree oils.	Topical, bath, room diffusion, inhalation, massage	• Madagascar, Australia • Steam • Leaves • Top	Use with caution in pregnancy.
Red Berry (Pepper, California) (*schinus molle*)	• Warm, woody-peppery, smoky scent. • Increases circulation, penetrating and soothing, reduces tension; helps to relieve discomfort loosens tight muscles. Stimulating, refreshing, balancing. Improves mental clarity. Helps breathing. • Blends well with black pepper, cinnamon, clove, and nutmeg.	Topical, bath, room diffusion, inhalation, massage	• South America, California • Steam • Berries • Middle	
Rosalina (*melaleuca ericifolia*)	• Soft medicinal, slightly woody floral scent. • Antiseptic, gentle expectorant with anti-infective properties. Useful in respiratory conditions, wounds, and infections. Calming, relaxing, and centering. • Blends well with citruses and other melaleucas.	Inhalation, massage, bath, room diffusion	• Australia • Steam • Leaves • Middle	

Essential Oil Common Name (*botanical name*)	Aroma Traditional and/or documented uses Blending	Methods of Use	Country of Origin Distillation Method Part of the Plant Note	Precautions
Rose, Cabbage Rose, Maroc (Absolute) (*rosa centifolia*)	• Deep, rich, sweet, floral scent. • Uplifting in times of emotional stress, grief, sadness, and depression. Aphrodisiac, nervine. Softening, purifying, and regenerative affect on the skin. Anti-inflammatory, applied locally to relieve itching. Useful in fertility and other female issues. Used extensively in perfumery. • Blends well with bergamot, clary sage, geranium, jasmine, lavender, neroli, palmarosa, patchouli, and sandalwood.	Topical, bath, inhalation, massage, perfume	• Morocco, Lebanon, Syria • Enfleurage, solvent extraction • Flowers • Middle	
Rose, Otto (*rosa damascena*)	• Soft and floral. Uplifting and tonifying. • Anti-inflammatory, neurotonic, sexual tonic. Antidepressant. Tonic effect on heart by activating sluggish blood circulation, relieving cardiac congestion and toning the capillaries. Soothes underlying tension and stress by releasing dopamine. Harmonizing for all skin types, but specific as a cell regenerator and moisturizer for mature and dry skin. Useful in fertility and other female issues. • Blends well with all oils.	Topical, bath, inhalation, massage, perfume	• Turkey, Bulgaria, Morocco, England • Steam • Flowers • Middle	

Rosemary (*rosemarinus officinalis*)	• Fresh, herbaceous and camphoric. • Neuromuscular relaxant, relieves tension. Improves poor circulation, eases and penetrates muscles, and helpful in rheumatic arthritis. Promotes digestion and aids in the assimilation of enzymes that breaks down food in the stomach. Helps the lymphatic system eliminate waste from the body; good for cellulite. Mucolytic, good respiratory and sinus disinfectant; useful for its clearing, energizing effects to inhalations and massage blends. Stimulating; helps memory, exhaustion, and alertness. • Blends well with basil, cedarwood, citruses, eucalyptus, frankincense, mints, myrtle, and ravensara.	Topical, bath, room diffusion, inhalation, massage	• Mediterranean, Spain, South France, Italy, Tunisia, Japan • Steam • Flowering tops and twigs • Middle	Not for asthmatics or epileptics. Can be too stimulating and may increase blood pressure. Use with caution in pregnancy.
Rosewood (Bois de Rose) (*aniba rosaeaodora*)	• Sweet, woody, floral scent. • An endangered plant...Use sparingly. Coriander seed is a good substitute. Balancing effect, boost to immune system. Restores libido. Mitigates effects of jet lag. Cell stimulant and tissue regenerator. Helps nervous tension, headaches, nausea, and stress-related disorders. • Blends well with citrus, floral, and wood oils.	Topical, room diffusion, bath, massage, perfume	• Brazil, Mexico • Steam • Tree bark • Middle	

Essential Oil Common Name (*botanical name*)	**Aroma Traditional and/or documented uses Blending**	**Methods of Use**	**Country of Origin Distillation Method Part of the Plant Note**	**Precautions**
Sage (*salvia officinalis*) Sage, Spanish (*salvia lavandulifolia*)	• Warm, herbaceous. • Antibacterial, antifungal, antiviral, anti-inflammatory. Dissolves lipids; useful against cellulite. Used to stimulate bile production. Strengthening, promotes digestion. Respiratory antiseptic and air purifier, mucolytic. Sage is known as an herb of wisdom, increasing intuition and self-awareness, purifies and clears unwanted energy from the person or environment. • Blends well with citruses, lavendin, and rosemary.	Topical, bath, room diffusion, inhalation, massage	• Mediterranean, China • Steam • Flowers and leaves • Middle	Topically, use in small quantities. Contains high ketone content-avoid use in epilepsy. Avoid in women with breast cancer and in pregnancy. Spanish sage is less toxic and safer to use.
Sandalwood (*santalum album*) Sandalwood, Australian (*santalum spicatum*)	• Soft, woody, sweet, and earthy. • An endangered plant in India.... Use sparingly. Cardiotonic, anti-infective. Useful for coughs, throat, and chest infections. Anti-inflammatory, antispasmodic; used for bladder infections. Useful for dry skin and acne. Relaxing, soothes nervous tension, and anxiety. Brings out emotions, helps one to dream; useful in meditation. A sexual tonic. Fixative in perfumes. • Blends well with benzoin, bergamot, citruses, coriander, jasmine, myrrh, and vetiver.	Topical, bath, inhalation, massage, perfume	• India, Indonesia, Australia • Heartwood • Steam • Base	

Savory, Mountain (*satureja montana*)	• Herbal, spicy, hot scent. • Analgesic, anti-infective, antiviral, antiparasitic. Circulatory tonic for hypotension. A neurotonic for nervous fatigue. Useful in rheumatoid arthritis, catarrh, colic, otitis, sclerosis, and spasm. • Blends well with citrus oils.	Topical, massage	• Europe, Asia • Steam • Whole plant • Middle	Use highly diluted in massage for fatigue or low energy. Use with caution in pregnancy.
Savory, Summer (*satureja hortense*)	• Fresh, herbaceous and spicy scent. • Improves circulation, relieves pain; use in low concentrations (1%) to warm muscles and benefit arthritis. Could be useful as an additive in treatments of any kind of infectious and fungal skin diseases. • Blends well with citruses, lavender, pine, and rosemary.	Topical, massage	• Europe, Asia • Steam • Whole plant • Middle	
Spanish Marjoram (*thymus mastichina*)	• Woody, sweet-herbal scent. • Upper respiratory decongestant, expectorant; helpful for cold and nasal congestion. Warming, improves circulation, dilates blood vessels. Relieves muscle aches, pains, painful menstruation, inflammation, and spasms. Improves digestion. A soothing nervine, relaxing, and calming. • Blends well with cedarwood, lavendin, oakmoss, pine, and rosemary.	Topical, bath, room diffusion, inhalation, massage	• Spain, Mediterranean area • Steam • Leaves • Middle	Avoid in pregnancy.

Essential Oil Common Name (*botanical name*)	Aroma Traditional and/or documented uses Blending	Methods of Use	Country of Origin Distillation Method Part of the Plant Note	Precautions
Spearmint (*mentha x spicata*)	• Sweet and minty, more mild than peppermint. • Stimulates a tired mind and helps with headaches, migraines, nervous strain, fatigue, and stress. Relaxes stomach muscles, relieves hiccups, nausea, and vomiting, flatulence, constipation, and diarrhea. Useful for pruritus. Good choice for children. • Blends well with benzoin, eucalyptus, lavender, lemon, other mints, and rosemary.	Topical, room diffusion, inhalation, massage	• Mediterranean, Europe, Russia, US • Steam • Leaves and flowering tops • Top	Avoid using before bedtime.
Spikenard (*nardostachys jatamansi*)	• Deep, earthy scent. • Most powerful sedative essential oil. Soothes stress and chronic insomnia. Restores balance to all skin types. Effective against dandruff, useful for psoriasis, and dry and itchy scalp. • Blends well with labdanum, lavender, oakmoss, patchouli, spice oils, and vetiver.	Topical, bath, inhalation, massage	• Asia • Steam • Root • Base	
Spruce, Hemlock (*tsuga canadensis*)	• Fresh, balsamic, sweet scent. • Useful for muscular aches and pains, asthma, coughs, and bronchitis. Reduces stress and anxiety, elevating, good for meditation. • Blends well with benzoin, cedarwood, lavender, pine, and rosemary.	Topical, room diffusion, bath, inhalation, massage	• North America • Bark and branches • Steam • Middle	

Tana (Issa) (*rhus tarantana*)	• Sharp, pungent, and balsamic. • Cooling, opens breathing. Reduces stress, refreshing. Mood uplifting, promotes alertness, helps to focus and concentrate, increases mental energy. Useful in the treatment of fatigue, stomach problems, and male sexual debility. There is some evidence that it could have cardiovascular activity, and supportive to the prostate. • Blends well with citrus and wood oils.	Topical, room diffusion, bath, inhalation, massage	• Madagascar • Steam • Whole plant • Middle to Top	
Tangerine (*citrus reticulata*)	• Light, sweet and cheerful. • Calming, sedating, helpful with stress, tension, anxiety, dizziness, and nervousness. Antispasmodic. Anti-inflammatory, anticoagulant. • Blends well with basil, chamomile, citruses, clary sage, chamomile, frankincense, and geranium.	Topical, bath, room diffusion, inhalation, massage	• Asia, US • Expressed • Peel • Top	Photosensitizing.
Tarragon (*artemisia dracunculus*)	• Herbal and anise-like scent. • Powerful neuromuscular spasmolytic. Antiviral. Has antiallergenic properties. One of the strongest antispasmodics, and is useful in colitis. Improves mental clarity and alertness. • Blends well with basil and lavender.	Topical, bath, room diffusion, inhalation, massage	• Russia • Steam • Whole plant • Middle	Avoid in glaucoma. Use in small amounts. Avoid in pregnancy.

Essential Oil Common Name (*botanical name*)	**Aroma Traditional and/or documented uses Blending**	**Methods of Use**	**Country of Origin Distillation Method Part of the Plant Note**	**Precautions**
Tea Tree (*melaleuca alternifolia*)	• Antiseptic, pungent, and fresh. • Broad spectrum antibacterial, antifungal, and antiviral. Immunostimulant. Reliable uses for bladder infection, candida overgrowth, and athlete's foot. A must for a first aid kit: use directly on burns, insect bites, nail fungus, cold sores, abrasions, abscesses, acne, or wherever there is sign of infection. Useful for fatigue. • Blends well with clove, eucalyptus, lavender, lemon, orange, and ravensara.	Topical, bath, room diffusion, inhalation, massage	• Australia, Tasmania • Steam • Leaves and twigs • Middle	
Thyme (*thymus vulgaris geraniol*)	• Sweet, green, herbaceous scent. • Antibacterial, antiviral, anti-yeast. Useful for upper respiratory and genital infections. Relieves intestinal distress caused by viral enteritis. • Blends well with lemon, lavender, orange, rosemary, and tea tree.	Topical, room diffusion, inhalation, massage	• Morocco, Spain, France, Greece, • Steam • Leaves, twigs • Middle	Can cause mild skin irritation. Avoid in pregnancy.
Thyme (*thymus vulgaris thujanol*)	• Warm, spicy, herbaceous scent. • Antiseptic. Useful for chlamydia and vaginitis. Stimulates the liver. • Blends well with bergamot, lemon, marjoram, pine, and rosemary.	Topical, room diffusion, inhalation, massage	• Morocco, Spain, France, Greece, • Steam • Leaves, twigs • Middle	Can cause mild skin irritation. Avoid in pregnancy.

Thyme Moroccan (*thymus satureioides*)	• Herbal and culinary scent. • Most effective essential oil for chronic infections and/or autoimmune diseases. Helps realign the immune system by reducing chronic inflammation caused by pathologically elevated levels of gamma globulins. • Blends well with bergamot, lemon, marjoram, pine, and rosemary.	Topical, room diffusion, inhalation, massage	• Morocco, Spain, France, Greece, Mediterranean Steam • Leaves, twigs • Middle	Can cause mild skin irritation. Avoid in pregnancy.
Thyme (*thymus vulgaris linalool*)	• Antiseptic aroma. • Systemic and topical anti-infective. Antiviral and antifungal; effective against candida albicans and staphylococcus (stomach, intestine, cystitis.) Tonic for nervous exhaustion. Excellent for impurities of the skin. • Blends well with bergamot, lemon, marjoram, pine, and rosemary.	Topical, room diffusion, inhalation, massage	• Morocco, Spain, France, Greece, Mediterranean • Steam • Leaves, twigs • Middle	Less irritating than other thymus species. Avoid in pregnancy.
Thyme, thymol type (*thymus vulgaris thymol*)	• Intensely herbal, stimulating, and energizing. • Broad anti-infective spectrum especially good against pathogenic bacteria and yeasts. Lifts depression caused by exhaustion and energizes. • Blends well with bergamot, lemon, marjoram, pine, and rosemary.	Topical, room diffusion, inhalation, massage	• Morocco, Spain, France, Greece, Mediterranean • Steam • Leaves, twigs • Middle	Dermocaustic. A skin irritant and should be used highly diluted. Avoid in high blood pressure. Avoid in pregnancy.

Essential Oil Common Name (*botanical name*)	Aroma Traditional and/or documented uses Blending	Methods of Use	Country of Origin Distillation Method Part of the Plant Note	Precautions
Tumeric (*curcuma longa*)	• Spicy, earthy, and woody. • Applied to the skin as a poultice to reduce pain and itching in small wounds. As a rubefacient, helpful for arthritis, rheumatism, and muscle aches and pains. Useful for flatulence and painful and sluggish digestion; may aid peptic ulcers. Relieves anxiety and stress. • Blends well with cassia, cinnamon, clary sage, ginger, labdanum, and ylang ylang.	Topical, inhalation, massage, perfumery	• South East Asia • Steam • Rhizome • Middle to base	Irritant in high concentrations. Avoid in pregnancy. Possible sensitizer.
Vanilla (*vanilla planifolia*)	• Rich, sweet, balsamic aroma. • Calming, warming, reduces stress; promotes a restful sleep. Mood uplifting, sensual, aphrodisiac. Helps one to dream. Antidepressant. Used extensively in perfumery. • Blends well with citrus, floral, spice, and wood oils.	Topical, bath, inhalation, massage, perfume	• Madagascar, Mexico, Central America • CO2, Solvent extraction • Unripe Pods • Base	
Vetiver (*vetiveria zizanioides*)	• Earthy, deep, smoky, and exotic aroma with sweet undertones. • Powerful circulatory and immunostimulant. Good for muscular aches. Provides sustained stimulation for endocrine glands. Comforting, sedating, and grounding; useful for stress and tension. Dilute in blends for acne and oily skin. Used as a fixative in perfumery, especially for men's colognes. • Blends well with citruses, jasmine, lavender, oakmoss, rose, rosemary, wood oils, and	Topical, bath, inhalation, massage, perfume	• Java, Indonesia, Philippines, Comoro Islands • Steam • Roots of the grass • Base	Avoid in pregnancy.

Wintergreen (*gaultheria fragrantissima*)	• Intense, sweet, fruity scent. • Refreshing and invigorating. Anti-inflammatory and analgesic, a counterirritant for rheumatoid arthritis. Used extensively in the flavoring industry. • Blends well with mints and citrus oils.	Room diffusion	• North America • Steam • Leaves • Middle to Top	Skin irritant in high dilutions. Always blend with other oils. Often adulterated with methyl salicylate. Avoid in pregnancy.
Yarrow (*achillea millefolium*)	• Soft herbal, camphorous aroma. • Anti-inflammatory, cell regenerating, analgesic. Applied externally for neuralgia or tendonitis. Improves catarrh. Improves mental clarity. • Blends well with cedarwood, chamomile, pine, and vetiver.	Topical, bath, inhalation, massage	• Europe, Asia, North America • Steam • Flowering plant • Middle	Contains ketones; Avoid in children less than 10 years old and in pregnancy. Avoid in epilepsy and asthma.
Ylang Ylang (*cananga odorata*)	• Extremely sweet, floral, and exotic. • Antispasmodic, relaxing, calms tachycardia and hypertension. Used as a muscle relaxant. Aphrodisiac, euphoric, and antidepressant. Aids irritability, nervousness, stress, anxiety, and depression. Helpful for oily skin. The first distillation is called Ylang Ylang Extra, which is the top grade. • Blends well with citrus oils, clary sage, jasmine, rose, spice oils, sandalwood, vetiver, and wood oils.	Topical, bath, inhalation, massage, perfume	• Comoros Islands, Java, Sumatra, Malaysia, Tahiti, India • Steam • Flowers • Middle to Base	

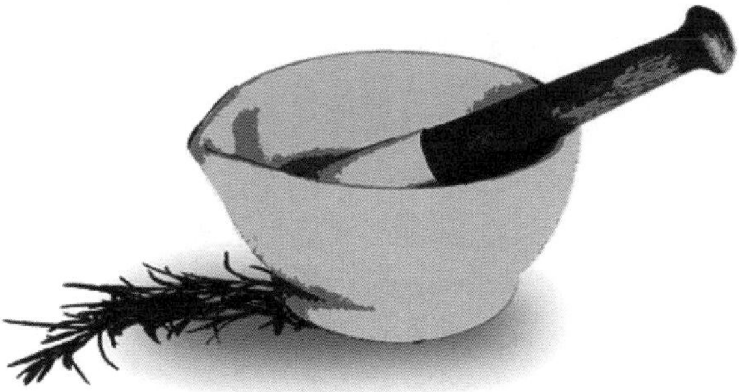

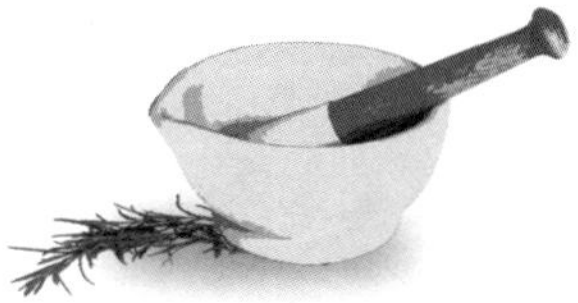

Carrier Oils

Because essential oils must be diluted prior to safe topical use, carrier oils are used. They are derived from seeds, nuts, kernels, fruits, and vegetables. Always look for "cold-pressed" carrier oils. This not only protects the delicate essential fatty acids (EFAs) from excessive heat, light and oxygen during processing and bottling, but "cold pressed" oils are 100% pure and contain more of the plant's natural ingredients. Other "refined" oils may contain petroleum residues from the solvents used in the extraction process that can remain in the oils and be absorbed by the skin.

Essential fatty acids are the building blocks of fats. There are two major types: linoleic (omega-6) and alpha-linolenic (omega-3). They function as essential building blocks in every membrane of every cell in the body, keeping beneficial substances within the cells and harmful ones out.

To keep carrier oils as fresh as possible, storage is recommended under refrigeration and in small containers. Only mix small amounts of aromatherapy products at any one time and use them quickly. It is also possible to extend the shelf life of carrier oils by adding small amount (less than 1%) of an antioxidant like Vitamin E or Grapefruit seed oils in the carrier oils.

The following chart describes some commonly used carrier oils. Any vegetable oil will work to dilute essential oils; some are preferred because of their therapeutic qualities.

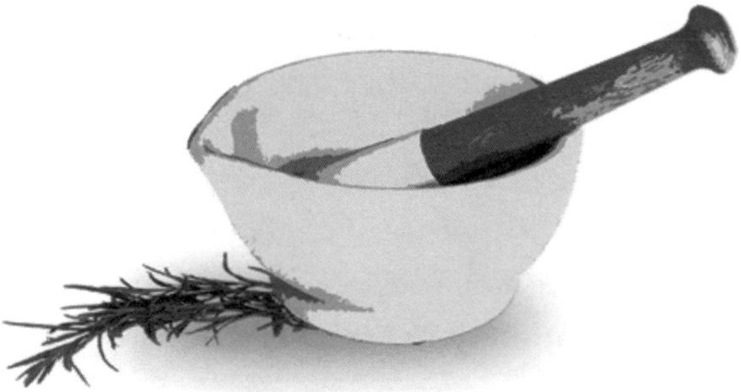

Carrier Oil Common Name (*botanical name*)	Description Traditional and/or documented uses and applications Shelf Life	Country of Origin Part of the Plant
Aloe Vera (*aloe barbadensis*)	• A pale, golden, odorless silky oil containing vitamins B1, B2, B6, C, niacinamide, choline and 18 amino acids. • Aloe vera oil is a moisturizer that has softening, healing, antimicrobial, and anti-inflammatory properties. Aloe vera penetrates the skin, supplying moisture directly to the tissue. It is effective in relieving thermal burn and sunburn, promoting new skin growth, and wound healing. Aloe vera gel is an astringent for normal to oily skin. • The shelf life is eight to twelve months.	• Africa, Asia, Europe, America • Leaf
Almond, Sweet (*prunus dulcis*)	• A light and fragrant oil. High in calcium, potassium, magnesium, iron, and phosphorus, and has a rich concentration of oleic and linoleic EFAs, beta-sitosterol, sqalene, and alpha–tocopherol. • Known to help repair the skin's lipid matrix barrier. An excellent emollient to help the skin balance the loss and absorption of moisture. Very lubricating, penetrates and softens the skin without leaving a greasy feeling. Not only does this oil help protect the skin's surface, but it also acts as a conditioner to help promote a clear, clean, young looking complexion. It helps relieve itching, irritation, inflammation, and soothes and moisturizes dry skin. Good for removing eye makeup. • Sweet almond oil has a shelf life of six months to a year.	• Asia, Mediterranean area • Nut of the tree
Apricot Kernal (*prunus armeniac*)	• A medium lightweight oil, quickly penetrating, non-greasy oil that is rich in oleic and linoleic EFAs and Vitamin A. • Suitable for a nourishing facial oil, especially for delicate, sensitive, inflamed, dry, or mature skin. Good for removing eye makeup. • The shelf life is six months to a year.	• Asia • Kernel of the fruit

Carrier Oil **Common Name** (***botanical name***)	**Description** **Traditional and/or documented uses and applications** **Shelf Life**	**Country of Origin** **Part of the Plant**
Arnica (*arnica montana*)	• A light, spicy, woodsy oil. • Arnica penetrates into the skin to help activate metabolism in underlying tissues. Traditionally, it has been used to promote burning of excessive fat deposits in the fat cells. The cleansing, nourishing, moisturizing, and lubricating action of Arnica oil helps improve overall skin conditions and appearance. Anti-inflammatory and analgesic; promotes healing of bruises and strains. Arnica increases blood flow to the area, without the warming effect of other counterirritants. Useful to potentiate other topical herbs—Mix with St. John's Wort Oil for nerve trauma. Do not use arnica on broken skin because it can cause irritation. Also good for treating the skin when it is chapped, cracked, or scaly. • The shelf life of Arnica oil depends on the base oil used in diffusion.	• Europe, Western North America • Flowers
Avocado (*persea gratissima*)	• An easily absorbed heavy oil, high in oleic acid and a good source of vitamins A, B1, B2, pantothenic acid, D and E, potassium, lecithin, amino acids, and sterols. • Avocado has the highest protein content of any fruit. It is said to mobilize and increase the collagen of connective tissue, and has been given the highest ranking by the Encyclopedia of Chemical Technology for sunscreen effectiveness. It is excellent for dry, mature, dehydrated, and wrinkled skin. Also used to treat sun or climate damaged skin that is dehydrated and under nourished, and for eczema and psoriasis. Good for massage oil, up to 20%, for added emolliency. Stored in cooler conditions, avocado oil can become cloudy, but will usually return to its normal color when it is again warmed. • The shelf life for refined avocado oil is between twelve to eighteen months, whereas the shelf life for crude avocado oil is six to nine months.	• Americas • Kernel and fruit of the tree
Baobab (*adansonia digitata*)	• Rich, golden oil has a high content of vitamins A, D, E, and oleic, linoleic, and linolenic fatty acids. • Baobab oil absorbs quickly, improves elasticity, and encourages regeneration of skin cells. It does not clog the pores. Said to alleviate pain from burns and regenerate the epithelial tissues in a short time, giving the skin tone and elasticity. Also used as an ingredient in formulations for eczema and psoriasis. • Baobab is highly stable oil with a shelf life of approximately two years.	• Africa, Australia, Madagascar • Seed/Fruit of the tree

Black Currant Seed (*ribes nigrum*)	• Considered one of the richest sources of gamma-linolenic acid (GLA), and has a high content of vitamin C and prostaglandins. • Black currant seed oil has a moderate immune-enhancing effect and reduces inflammation. It is often combined with vitamin E to prevent oxidation. It is good for general skin care, and is soothing and healing. In massage oil, it can be mixed up to 20%. Excess use may result in oily skin, an indication to decrease dosage. • The shelf life is six months to a year.	• Europe, Asia • Seeds of the plant
Borage (*borago officinalis*)	• Light and sweet with a thin to medium texture. • Penetrates skin easily, and leaves a mildly oily feel. It is high in GLA that helps inhibit the skin's aging process; encourages skin and tissue regeneration, and reduces inflammation. Borage oil has also been used for eczema and other chronic skin conditions, and especially dry, dehydrated, mature, or aging skin. Borage oil is usually blended in a small (10-20%) dilution with other carrier oils. • Borage oil has an average shelf life of three to six months if properly stored and kept refrigerated.	• Mediterranean area • Seeds of the plant
Calendula (*calendula officinalis*)	• A thick oil with a high content and diversity of carotenes, phytosterols, polyphenols, EFAs, and vitamin A. • It is a toning soothing, restorative oil, good for any type of skin, but especially suitable for dry skin. It helps preserve skin freshness, protect skin from dehydration, sun-induced wrinkles, and sun damage. When used regularly the oil imparts deep olive shine to the skin, and helps prctect skin from age related thinning and drying. It is best when infused in a light textured oil such as almond or sunflower. Traditionally, it has been used to prevent tearing, soothe pain, stop bleeding, promote rapid healing, and prevent scarring. • The shelf life of calendula oil depends on the base oil in which it was infused.	• Europe, US • Infused Flowers

Carrier Oil **Common Name** (*botanical name*)	**Description** **Traditional and/or documented uses and applications** **Shelf Life**	**Country of Origin** **Part of the Plant**
Calophyllum (Tamanu) (*calophyllum inophyllum*)	• Research shows that this oil contains three basic classes of lipids: neutral lipids, glycolipids, and phospholipids. • The oil also contains a unique fatty acid called calophyllic acid, and a novel antibiotic lactone and non-steroidal anti-inflammatory agent called calophyllolide. These and other components of calophyllum oil, including anti-inflammatory coumarins, account for some of the oil's beneficial activity as an antibacterial and anti-inflammatory. It possesses a unique capacity to promote the formation of new tissue, thereby accelerating wound healing and the growth of healthy skin; this process is known as cicatrization. Traditionally, it can be applied liberally to cuts, scrapes, burns, insect bites and stings, abrasions, acne and acne scars, psoriasis, diabetic sores, anal fissures, sunburn, dry or scaly skin, blisters, eczema, herpes sores, and athletes foot. Also reduces foot and body odor. • The shelf life is six months to a year.	• Southeast Asia, Madagascar • Kernel of the fruit
Canola (Rapeseed) (*brassica napus*)	• This quickly penetrating, medium light oil contains a high linoleic acid content, vitamin E, and minerals. • This oil is considered to be a good moisturizer and healing agent and can be used in place of more expensive products. Works well in massage oils. • Has a three to six month shelf life if kept properly in airtight container. Refrigerate after opening.	• Canada • Pods/Seeds of the plant
Camellia (*camellia sasanqua*)	• One of the most rapidly absorbed oils, it contains vitamins, A, B, and E, and the minerals phosphorus calcium, iron, manganese, and magnesium. • Camellia helps maintain the nature of the skin, and to prevent formation of such skin disorders as wrinkles, freckles, and acne. It helps to restructure the skin and strengthen nails. Given these properties, it is a good active ingredient in nourishing shampoos and lotions for dry, damaged and delicate hair and after-sun products for thin and normal hair; emollient gels for around the eyes; softening hand creams; restructuring creams for damaged skin; moisturizing creams for dry skin; and products for normal and mature skin. • The shelf life is six months to a year and should be stored in a dark, cool area.	• Japan • Seed of the plant

Carrot Root (*daucus carota*)	• Rejuvenating, moisturizing, and nourishing and high in minerals, beta-carotene, and vitamin A. • It is used for prematurely aging and dry, itchy skin, acne skin conditions, dermatitis, skin irritation, skin rashes, and wrinkles. Good for massage oil, up to 20%. Carrot seed oil is an essential oil and must be diluted prior to use. • The shelf life is one year.	• Mediterranean area, Afghanistan • Root of the plant
Cocoa Butter (*theobroma cacao*)	• A tan colored butter with pleasant cocoa odor, and used in a variety of cosmetic, toiletry, and pharmaceutical applications. • Cocoa butter is used to reduce cutaneous dryness and improve skin flexibility. It is also used as a skin and hair moisturizer. In soaps, cocoa butter is used to harden soaps and is a rich moisturizer. • Cocoa butter has an almost indefinite shelf life.	• Central America • Beans of the tree
Coconut (*cocos nucifera*)	• A light and penetrating oil that, when used in soaps, makes abundant rich creamy lather. • Coconut oil is widely used in hair care, particularly well suited to scalp treatments. Very soothing and nourishing on dry skin. Helps with stretch marks. Useful in making ointments. • The shelf life is over one year if kept in a cool place.	• Southeast Asia, Philippines Seeds/Nut of the tree
Evening Primrose (*oenothera biennis*)	• A fine textured, nourishing, and emollient oil with superb moisturizing properties containing high amounts of linoleic, linolenic, arachidonic, and GLA. • Evening primrose is known to promote normal cell growth. It is effective in helping with eczema, psoriasis, PMS, rheumatoid arthritis, and weight reduction. It can reduce hyperactivity in babies and young children when rubbed onto their skin. It promotes healthy skin, helps clear skin blemishes, soothe irritations, and softens wrinkles exaggerated by dryness. Good for massage oil, up to 20%. • Evening primrose oil does not have a very long shelf life and should be stored accordingly. Keep away from light and heat.	• Europe • Seeds of the plant

Carrier Oil **Common Name** (***botanical name***)	**Description** **Traditional and/or documented uses and applications** **Shelf Life**	**Country of Origin** **Part of the Plant**
Flaxseed (*linum usitatissimum*)	• A rich, yellow color oil containing 15-25% linoleic acid, 50-60% linolenic acid, vitamin E, lecithin, all of the essential amino acids, and almost every trace mineral. • It regulates skin permeability, promotes cell regeneration, and restructures and moisturizes skin. It is useful for preventing scarring and stretch marks. This oil is prone to rancidity and should be kept away from heat and light. • Shelf life is approximately three to six months with proper storage.	• US • Seeds of the plant
Grapeseed (*vitis vinifera*)	• A non-greasy light oil that absorbs and spreads easily. Contains vitamins, minerals, and protein, a small amount of vitamin E, and is rich in linoleic acid, necessary for normal cell growth. • Grapeseed oil has regenerative, restructuring, and superior moisturizing attributes. Blending with another carrier oil such as sweet almond or wheat germ oil often enriches it. Grapeseed is ideal for use in products for thin, greasy, damaged, and delicate hair. Useful in body hygiene creams, lip balms, hand creams, and regenerative products for mature, damaged, and stressed skin, notably for use around the eyes and neck. It is slightly astringent, thus tightens and tones the skin. Store in a cool, dark area. • The shelf life is six months to a year if kept properly in airtight container.	• Asia • Seeds of the fruit
Hazelnut (*corylus avellana*)	• Lubricating and nourishing, contains high amounts of linoleic acid, vitamins, minerals, and protein. • It has been used to tone and tighten the skin while strengthening capillaries and assisting in cell regeneration. Has good astringent qualities which makes it useful for oily or combinations skins and acne. It stimulates cell regeneration, repairs dry and damaged skin, tones and tightens the skin, and helps maintain firmness and elasticity. • Has a shelf life of six months to a year if kept properly in airtight container.	• Europe, Asia • Nut/kernel of the tree

Hemp (*cannabis sativa*)	• An easily penetrating and moisturizing oil derived from the non-narcotic variety of plant. It has a perfect 3:1 ratio of omega-6: omega-3 EFAs, 56.9% linoleic acid, 18.9% linolenic acid, and 1.7% gamma-linolenic acid. Hemp oil also contains the natural anti-oxidant vitamin E and sterols. • Hemp revives and repairs cells damaged by the sun, wind, and ultraviolet light and may play a preventive role in the skin aging process. It may be used as a massage oil to help soothe muscles. It may also be added to shampoo or conditioner to rejuvenate the scalp. • Hemp oil is prone to rancidity and should be properly stored or used right away. In the refrigerator, the shelf life is about twelve months.	• Canada • Seed of the plant
Jojoba (*simmondsia chinensis*)	• A liquid wax that is extremely stable and does not easily deteriorate. It is rich in Vitamin E and contains myristic acid. • The structure of jojoba oil closely resembles that of the skin's sebum. Its anti-inflammatory actions make it useful for psoriasis, dermatitis, and acne problems. It helps dissolve sebum and unclog pores. Jojoba penetrates skin rapidly to soften and moisturize skin of all types. Especially useful for dry, mature, aging skin, wrinkles, and stretch marks. It is frequently blended with other carrier oils for massage oil, up to 50%. • It has the longest shelf life of all the carrier oils, well over two years.	• US, Mexico • Beans of the shrub
Kukui Nut (*aleurites moluccana*)	• A very light oil, transparent, low-viscosity oil containing. Contains vitamins A, C and E, all antioxidants and 19%oleic, 41% lincleic, and less than 27% linolenic acid. • It moisturizes without being greasy. Kukui nut oil is quickly absorbed may be used on all skin types. It is considered to be beneficial for balancing, softening, and rejuvenating the skin. Good for dry skin, eczema, psoriasis, sunburn, and acne. • Kukui nut oil goes rancid rather quickly, within six months.	• Asia, Hawaii • Nut of the tree

Carrier Oil **Common Name** (*botanical name*)	**Description** **Traditional and/or documented uses and applications** **Shelf Life**	**Country of Origin** **Part of the Plant**
Macadamia Nut (*macadamia integrifolia*)	• A thick, readily absorbed oil, clear in color with a slight tinge of yellow. Contains high amounts of palmitoleic acid, which is also normally found in our own skin's sebum. • Macadamia nut is very emollient and is therefore good for dry, mature, and aging skin, where sebum production has decreased. Macadamia oil has been used to help reduce fine lines when included in a facial massage blend. It also leaves an oil film on the skin and, if not carefully used or used in a small dilution with another carrier oil, it may overpower a blend. • The shelf life is one year.	• Australia • Nut of the tree
Meadowfoam (*limnanthes alba*)	• A light, stable, non-greasy, high quality moisturizing, and rapidly absorbed oil, made up of 97% very long chain fatty acids (C20 and C22). • It is one of the most moisturizing oils for skin and hair and provides a protective barrier. It is long lasting, and reduces the effect of aging on the skin. It has excellent uses with other cosmetic oils. • The long chains make the oil particularly stable and resistant to oxidation and deterioration. It is 20 times more stable than soybean oil. The shelf life is 2 years or more.	• Northwest US • Flowers
Neem (*azadirachta indica*)	• The main constituent in neem oil is azadirachtin consisting of over 40 different liminoids, with steroid like properties. It is rich in fatty acids and glycerides and contains sulfur compounds that contribute to the pungent odor. • Neem provides an excellent natural moisturizing base for skin care formulations. A natural antifungal, antibacterial, and antiviral oil, useful for bruises, cuts, and skin disorders. This oil has been used for centuries in traditional Indian medicine to aid in the healing of topical skin disorders such as eczema, psoriasis, rashes, burns, and acne. Use up to 10% in skin and hair care products and soaps. • The shelf life is approximately two years if kept in a cool place.	• Asia, India • Seeds of the tree

Palm (*elaeisis guineensis*)	• Palm oil is rich in vitamin E and is one of the richest natural plant sources of carotenes. • Used extensively for its emollient properties. Palm oil is also less drying than coconut oil, but if used in excess, palm kernel oil can also be drying to the skin. It softens the skin, protects it against damage, promotes healing, and gives it a more youthful, healthy appearance. • This oil has an excellent shelf life of two years.	• Africa • Kernels/Seeds and fruit of the tree
Peanut (*arachis hypogaea*)	• A clear, thick oil, light in aroma with a slight fatty, nutty quality. Contains a high content of vitamin E. • It is regarded as non-drying, conditioning oil, similar to olive and castor oils. Non-penetrating and leaves a very oily film on the skin, thereby making it a good choice for inclusion in massage blends. It is best used to dilute stronger smelling essential oils. It is good for all skin types, and is an emollient for arthritis or sunburn. It also strengthens weak and brittle nails. Peanut oil is said to increase the blood circulation after treatment, the skin will feel warm and have a reddish glow. • The shelf life is six months to one year.	• US, Central and South America • Nuts of the plant
Pistachio Nut (*pistacia vera*)	• A light, rapidly absorbed, non-greasy oil, rich in iron, potassium, calcium, phosphorous, and folic acid. • Although it can be relatively expensive, pistachio nut oil can be combined with other carrier oils. It is an excellent emollient and provides moisture to the skin. Pistachio oil compares favorably to peanut oil and will soften and nourish the skin. • The shelf life of Pistachio nut oil is three to six months.	• Asia • Nut of the tree
Pumpkin Seed (*cucurbita pepo*)	• A heavier carrier oil, high in protein, zinc, and polyunsaturated fats that exhibit antioxidant activity and anti-inflammatory properties. • Traditionally it has been used for skin problems such as sores and ulcers. It makes a good massage oil blend when mixed up to 20% with another carrier oil. • The shelf life is one year.	• Americas • Seeds of the plant

Carrier Oil Common Name (*botanical name*)	**Description Traditional and/or documented uses and applications Shelf Life**	**Country of Origin Part of the Plant**
Rose Hip Seed (Rosa Mosqueta) (*rosa rubiginosa*)	• Mild, earthy, and easily absorbed. Rose hip seed oil contains trans-Retinoic acid, a derivative of retinol (Vitamin A). It is high in linoleic and linolenic acids. • Rose Hip Seed oil has recently been used to help reduce the signs of aging (especially the fine lines around the eyes and mouth) and the drying effects of the sun and climate. It is an exceptional skin nutrient and emollient, assist with healing of scars, burns, softening of keloids, and smoothing of stretch marks. It is included in face moisturizers and body creams, and is ideal for all skin types. It is usually blended in a small (often 10%) dilution with other carrier oils. • It goes rancid rather quickly, within six months. Best stored in a cool place.	• Mediterranean area • Hips and seeds of the bush
Safflower (*carthamus tinctorius*)	• A light, easily spreadable oil, high in linoleic acid, having superior skin compatibility. • It increases the moisture content of the skin. Safflower oil makes a suitable base, but it is recommended to mix other carrier oils (especially those with good antioxidant qualities). Useful for moisturizing all skin types and may be beneficial for painful, inflamed joints, arthritis, bruises, and sprains. • Because safflower oil goes rancid quickly, having a shelf life of less than three months, it can be mixed with another carrier oil to increase the shelf life.	• India • Seeds of the plant
Sea Buckthorn (*hippophae rhamnoides*)	• This oil is golden-red in color and has thick consistency. It contains vitamins A, K, E, C, B1, B2, folic acid, amino acids, and minerals. It is a rich source of linoleic and linolenic acid in 1:1 ratio, and in palmitic and palmitoleic acids. It is also a powerful antioxidant due to high phytochemical content, which includes carotenoids, flavonoids, and phytosterols. • Sea buckthorn oil is an indispensable ingredient in restorative, anti-aging, and revitalizing skin care. It is an excellent natural UV (B-range) protector. It is used specifically to help damaged skin, ulcerations, scar tissue, wrinkles, eczema, and burns. Recent studies show that Sea buckthorn oil enhances microcirculation and epidermal regeneration. It is very concentrated oil and therefore dilution of sea buckthorn oil with any lighter carrier oil is recommended. • The shelf life is one year.	• Europe, Asia • Berries of the shrub

Sesame (*sesamum indicum*)	• A thick oil, considered to be strong smelling. A good source of vitamins E and B complex, and minerals such as calcium, magnesium, and phosphorus, proteins, and lecithin, and high oleic and linoleic acids. • Sesame oil is a natural skin moisturizer, and used for eczema, psoriasis, and mature skin. It is best mixed with another carrier oil, such as almond or grapeseed to make it a bit lighter. Good choice for massage therapists as it does not stain sheets. It is best used to dilute stronger smelling essential oils. • The shelf life is one year.	• Africa, Asia, India • Seeds of the plant
Shea Butter (*butyrosperum parkii*)	• This plant butter is high in triglycerides, fatty acids, and vitamins A and E. • An excellent moisturizer for all skin types. It penetrates deeply to help skin regain elasticity, repairs scar tissue, eases sun burn, reduces wrinkles, and adds moisture to dry hair. Some clinical observations suggest that Shea Butter increases local blood circulation in the skin, improving the elimination of waste products. Other studies suggest that Shea Butter helps to improve the elasticity of the skin, making it a valuable addition to products for all skin types. • Store at room temperature in amber for approximately two years.	• Africa • Nut kernels of the tree
Soybean (*soja hispida*)	• A light oil, easily absorbed, with a mild aroma. Contains 2% lecithin, proteins, vitamin C, A, E, and K. Rich in phytoestrogens, and oleic, linoleic, and linolenic EFAs. • It nourishes all skin types, and is a strong emollient. It is susceptible to oxidation and can be a skin sensitizer. • The shelf life is one year.	• Asia • Bean of the plant
St. John's Wort (*hypericum perforatum*)	• An infused oil containing hypericin like compounds, bioflavonoids, polyphenols, monoterpens, phytosterols, EFAs, and other nutrients. • It is nourishing to the skin, especially sensitive skin. It is a valuable anti-inflammatory that can help speed the healing of wounds, bruises, varicose veins, sunburns, bee stings, and mild burns. Traditionally used to promote recovery of skin and mucous injuries. Helps combat bacterial infections, reverses inflammation, and reduces skin itching and irritability. It may induce hypersensitivity to sunlight. • The shelf life is approximately one year.	• Europe • Whole plant

Carrier Oil **Common Name** (*botanical name*)	**Description** **Traditional and/or documented uses and applications** **Shelf Life**	**Country of Origin** **Part of the Plant**
Sunflower (*helianthus annuus*)	• A very lightweight and easily absorbable oil. Contains EFAs and a high amount of vitamin E. • It is inexpensive and can be blended with a variety of other carrier oils; however, is not as suitable for massage due to the absorption rate (unless blended with other carrier oils). It is good for all skin types and helpful for dry and delicate skin. • Shelf life is approximately three to six months.	• US • Seeds of the plant
Vitamin E	• A very thick oil which is high in antioxidants. • Vitamin E extends the shelf life of other carrier oils and natural aromatherapy products. Vitamin E penetrates below the skin's surface and is used for healing effects on wounds and its ability to retard the conversion of soluble collagen to insoluble collagen, thereby reducing the chance of scar tissue formation. It rejuvenates damaged skin cells and promotes healthy regeneration of scarred skin. Vitamin E may help the skin overcome the harmful effects of the sun. It helps to preserve the health and integrity of the skin, and helps in the healing of cuts, abrasions and post surgical scar tissue. It provides a defense against bacterial infection, promotes cellular oxygenation, and protects and insulates the skin from premature signs of aging. It prevents scarring and may fade existing scars with regular use. Look for 100% alpha-tocopherol oil. • It has a shelf life of two years or more.	• USA • Wheat, Corn, Soy or Canola

Walnut (*juglans regia*)	• An unsaturated, easily absorbed, light oil. Contains phosphorous, iron, calcium, magnesium, potassium, copper, and polyunsaturated fatty acids. • Walnut oil has astringent properties and is a good emollient and moisturizing oil, with anti-aging, regenerative, and toning properties. This oil has many benefits when used in the healing of wounds and skin problems such as eczema, herpes, psoriasis, and skin parasites. It can be used for all skin types in anti-wrinkle products and creams for dry, normal, and mature skin, body and hygiene products, massage blends, and lip balms. • It has a shelf life of six months to one year.	• America, Europe, Asia • Nuts of the tree
Wheatgerm (*tritcum vulgare*)	• A thick, strong oil, rich in naturally occurring antioxidants including vitamins E and B1, beta carotene, proteins, and phosphatides, phytosterols, and 58% linoleic acid. • It is often added to other carriers to help lengthen their shelf life to prevent rancidity. Traditionally, it is used to promote a smoother, younger looking skin, and assist in healing scar tissue and stretch marks. It is nourishing to dry, cracked, or mature skin, and helps promote the formation of new cells, and improves circulation. It helps repair sun damage to the skin. It is also used to soothe eczema and psoriasis. It works well in a massage oil blend when mixed up to 10% with another carrier oil. • If kept properly in airtight container, its shelf life is 12 to 18 months. Should be refrigerated after opening.	• USA • Grain of the plant

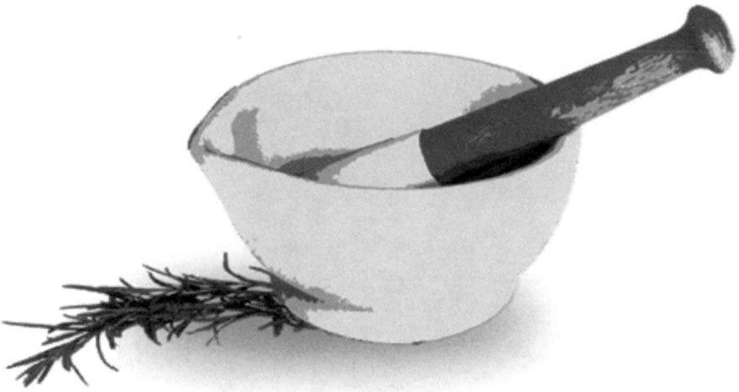

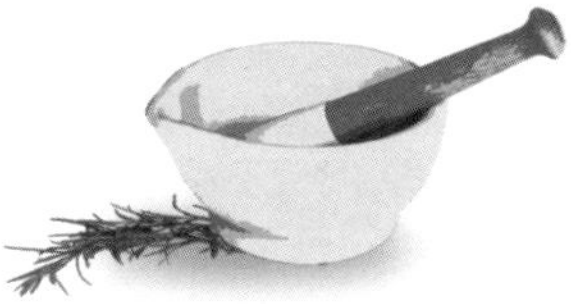

Condition Reference Guide

Holistic medicine and aromatherapy look at the whole person—physical, emotional, spiritual, lifestyle—in determining a "treatment" for various symptoms. In the absence of a practitioner, below are listed some common ailments for which essential oil use is well suited.

Condition	Essential Oil	Method of Use
Abdominal Cramps/ Indigestion	Allspice, Anise, Basil, Cardamom, Caraway, Coriander, Dill, Fennel, Ginger, Lemon, Mandarin, Sweet Marjoram, Nutmeg, Orange, Peppermint	Massage, bath, topical as localized rub diluted in oil/lotion
Acne	Bergamot, Blue Cypress, Cajeput, Calendula, Camellia, Carrot Seed and Root, Cedarwood, Geranium, Roman Chamomile, Hazelnut, Jojoba, Juniper, Kanuka, Kukui, Lavender, Lemon, Lemon Scented Tea Tree, Myrtle, Neem, Niaouli, Palmarosa, Petitgrain, Rosemary, Tea Tree	Topically as a face tonic, wash, or diluted oil
Allergy	Blue Cypress, Chamomile, Eucalyptus, Hyssop, Niaouli, Lavender, Melissa	Inhalation, bath, room diffusion, massage
Antibacterial	Clove, Eucalyptus, Lavender, Lemon Myrtle, Marjoram, Oregano, Palmarosa, Rosemary, Sage, Savory, Tea Tree, Thyme	Topical, bath, spritzer
Anxiety	Basil, Cedarwood, Chamomile, Geranium, Lavender, Lemon Verbena, Mandarin, Myrrh, Neroli, Orange, Patchouli, Petitgrain, Rose, Vetiver, Ylang Ylang	Inhalation, massage, bath, perfume, room diffusion

Condition	Essential Oil	Method of Use
Arthritis/ Tendonitis	Arnica, Birch, Black Pepper, Cajuput, Chamomile, Eucalyptus, Helichrysum, Juniper, Lavender, Lemon, Yarrow	Massage, compress, bath, concentrated rub
Athlete's Foot/ Fungus Infections	Blue Cypress, Chamomile, Cinnamon, Clove, Kanuka, Kunzea, Lavender, Manuka, Niaouli, Oregano, Peppermint, Sage, Savory, Tea Tree, Thyme	Topical as a spray, foot bath, or diluted oil
Bruises	Aloe Vera, Arnica, Helichrysum, Calendula, Callophylum, Chamomile, Hyssop, Sweet Marjoram, Lavender, St John's Wort	Topical as a diluted oil, spray, or compress
Burns	Blue Cypress, Calophyllum, Chamomile, Geranium, Lavender (neat), Rose Hip Seed	Compress/ dressing, diluted spray
Cellulite	Arnica, Cedarwood, Cypress, Eucalyptus, Fennel, Geranium, Juniper, Lavender, Lemon, Lemongrass, Niaouli, Rosemary, Sage	Massage, bath, herbal wrap
Circulation	Basil, Black Spruce, Cedarwood, Cinnamon, Coriander, Cypress, Eucalyptus, Geranium, Ginger, Juniper, Peppermint, Petitgrain, Pine, Rosemary, Sage	Massage, bath
Coughs	Cedarwood, Roman Chamomile, Cypress, Eucalyptus, Geranium, Lemon, Sweet Marjoram, Peppermint, Pine, Ravensara	Inhalation, room diffusion, topical rub
Cuts/Scrapes/ Wounds	Chamomile, Cypress, Geranium, Helichrysum, Lavender, Lemon, Niaouli, Rosemary, Tea Tree	Topical spray
Depression	Bergamot, Clary Sage, Geranium, Jasmine, Melissa, Neroli, Peppermint, Pine, Rose, Sandalwood, Ylang Ylang	Inhalation, massage, bath, room diffusion, perfume
Disinfectants	Eucalyptus, Grapefruit, Lemon, Nerolina, Pine, Sage	Topical
Energy/Fatigue	Basil, Black Spruce, Cedarwood, Clove, Eucalyptus, Ginger, Hyssop, Juniper, Lemon, Peppermint, Pine, Rosemary, Savory, Tana, Tea Tree	Inhalation, massage, bath, room diffusion, perfume

Condition	Essential Oil	Method of Use
Fluid Retention/ Edema	Cedarwood, Cypress, Geranium, Juniper, Lavender, Lemongrass, Pine, Rosemary, Tea Tree	Bath, massage
Hair/Scalp	Chamomile, Lavender, Lavender Spike, Rosemary, Ylang Ylang	Topical in a shampoo, or diluted oil
Headache	Anise, Roman Chamomile, Lavender, Lemon, Sweet Marjoram, Peppermint, Rosemary	Inhalation, massage, bath, room diffusion
Immune Support	Bay Laurel, Eucalyptus, Geranium, Lavender, Lemon Myrtle, Palmarosa, Pine, Ravensara, Rosemary, Tea Tree	Inhalation, bath, massage, room diffusion
Indigestion/ Heartburn	Anise Basil, Cardamom, Coriander, Dill, Fennel, Ginger, Orange, Black Pepper, Peppermint, Rosemary	Massage, compress, topical rub
Insect Bites	Basil, Blue Cypress, Cajuput, Calophyllum, Chamomile, Lavender, Niaouli, Tea Tree	Topical spray, diluted oil
Insomnia	Roman Chamomile, Lavender, Lemon Verbena, Mandarin, Sweet Marjoram, Melissa, Neroli, Orange, Sandalwood, Spikenard, Ylang Ylang	Massage, bath, room diffusion, 1-2 drops on pillow
Meditation	Buddha Wood, Blue Cypress, Frankincense, Myrrh, Patchouli, Sandalwood, Spikenard, Vetiver	Inhalation, room diffusion, perfume
Menopause	Clary Sage, Cypress, Fennel, Frankincense, Geranium, Lavender, Mandarin, Melissa, Rose	Bath, room diffusion, massage, spritzer
Menstrual Cramps	Anise, Roman Chamomile, Clary Sage, Lavender, Lemon Verbena, Mandarin Sweet Marjoram, Yarrow	Massage, bath, compress, sitz bath
Muscle Aches/ Strains/ Sports Injuries	Arnica, Birch, Black Pepper, Calendula, Chamomile, Eucalyptus, Ginger, Helichrysum, Juniper, Kanuka, Lemon Scented Tea Tree, Manuka, Sweet Marjoram, Nutmeg, Rosemary, St. John's Wort	Massage, concentrated rub, bath, compress
Nausea/ Motion Sickness	Caraway, Clove, Coriander, Fennel, Ginger, Mandarin, Black Pepper, Peppermint, Sandalwood, Spearmint	Inhalation, room diffusion, massage

Condition	Essential Oil	Method of Use
PMS	Bergamot, Clary Sage, Geranium, Grapefruit, Jasmine, Mandarin, Neroli, Rose, Sage, Ylang Ylang	Bath, massage, room diffusion
Rashes/ Dermatitis	Blue Cypress, Chamomile, Evening Primorse, Geranium, Helichrysum, Jojoba, Juniper, Lavender, Lemon, Palmarosa, Rose, Sandalwood, Tea Tree	Bath, compress, topical as a spritzer or concentrated oil/lotion
Respiratory	Arina, Basil, Cajeput, Cypress, Cedarwood, Elemi, Eucalyptus, Fir, Hyssop, Lantana, Lavender, Lemon, Lemon Myrtle, Nerolina, Niaouli, Pine, Sweet Marjoram, Ravensara, Rosalina, Rosemary, Sage	Inhalation, bath, massage, room diffusion
Scars	Cedarwood, Calophyllum, Carrot Seed, Galbanum, Helichrysum, Labdanum, Lavender, Neroli, Sage	Topical as a concentrated oil/lotion
Shingles	Blue Cypress, Calophyllum, Chamomile, Clove Bud, Geranium, Ravensara, Sage, Thyme	Bath, compress, spritzer
Stress Relief/ Nervous Tension	Benzoin, Bergamot, Cedarwood, Chamomile, Clary Sage, Jasmine, Geranium, Grapefruit, Lavender, Lemon Verbena, Mandarin, Sweet Marjoram, Melissa, Neroli, Orange, Patchouli, Petitgrain, Rose, Black Spruce, Tangerine, Vetiver, Ylang Ylang	Inhalation, bath, massage, room diffusion, perfume
Sunburn	Chamomile, Eucalyptus radiata, Geranium, Lavender, Sandalwood	Bath, compress, spritzer
Varicose Veins	Basil, Bay Laurel, Calendula, Calophyllum, Clary Sage, Cypress, Neroli, Niaouli, Lavender, Lemon, Rose Hip Seed	Bath, concentrated rub, compress
Warts	Blue Cypress, Clove, Manuka, Oregano, Tea Tree, Thyme	Compress, concentrated application

As a quick reference, the following charts list some easy to locate essential oils and carrier oils for common skin care conditions.

Essential Oils	Baby skin	Blemished skin	Chapped skin	Dehydrated Skin	Dry Skin	Eczema, dry	Eczema, moist	Facial Lines	General skin care	Healing	Inflamed Skin	Mature/ Aging skin	Moisturizing	Normal skin	Oily skin	Psoriasis	Scars	Sensitive skin	Stretch Marks	Wrinkles
Basil						•									•					
Cedarwood		•			•				•					•	•					
Chamomile, German		•				•	•										•	•		
Chamomile, Roman	•	•			•	•	•							•		•	•	•		
Clary Sage		•							•			•			•					
Cypress								•				•			•	•				•
Eucalyptus		•					•								•		•			
Frankincense					•		•	•		•	•	•					•	•	•	•
Geranium		•		•	•				•			•		•	•		•			
Jasmine					•				•			•						•		
Juniper		•					•								•		•			

Essential Oils	Baby skin	Blemished skin	Chapped skin	Dehydrated Skin	Dry Skin	Eczema, dry	Eczema, moist	Facial Lines	General skin care	Healing	Inflamed Skin	Mature/ Aging skin	Moisturizing	Normal skin	Oily skin	Psoriasis	Scars	Sensitive skin	Stretch Marks	Wrinkles
Lavender	•	•	•		•	•	•		•	•		•		•	•		•	•	•	
Lemon		•				•	•		•					•	•	•				
Myrrh									•			•								
Neroli								•	•								•	•	•	•
Niaouli							•													
Orange	•								•					•						
Palmarosa						•			•											
Patchouli		•	•		•		•					•					•			
Rose	•				•				•			•		•	•			•		
Rosemary		•												•	•		•		•	
Rosewood					•				•											
Sandalwood		•	•	•	•	•			•		•	•		•	•		•	•	•	
Tea Tree		•													•					
Ylang Ylang		•			•				•			•		•	•					

Skin Care Uses with Carrier Oils

Carrier Oils	Baby skin	Blemished skin	Chapped skin	Dehydrated Skin	Dry Skin	Eczema, dry	Eczema, moist	Facial Lines	General skin care	Healing	Inflamed Skin	Mature/ Aging skin	Moisturizing	Normal skin	Oily skin	Psoriasis	Scars	Sensitive skin	Stretch Marks	Wrinkles
Almond	•	•							•	•	•		•	•						
Apricot			•		•						•	•		•				•		
Avocado					•	•						•				•				•
Borage			•	•	•	•					•	•								
Calophyllum		•				•	•			•	•					•				
Canola													•							
Evening Primrose	•	•				•	•	•								•	•			•
Grapeseed												•	•		•					
Hazelnut	•	•				•			•			•								
Jojoba		•	•		•			•					•	•		•	•		•	•
Rose Hip Seed			•		•			•		•		•		•					•	•
Sesame							•					•				•				
Shea Butter					•				•	•			•	•	•					•
Vitamin E										•		•					•			

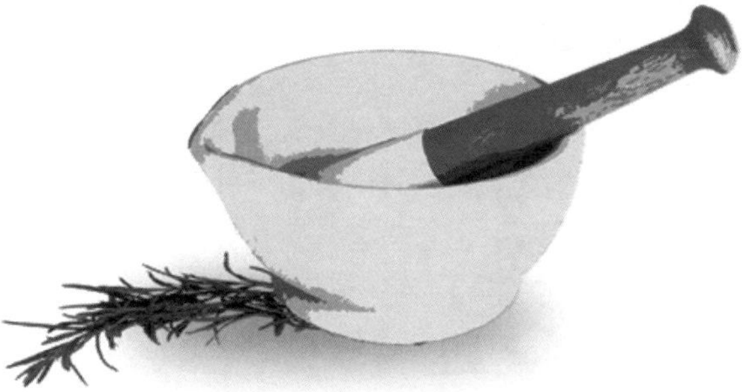

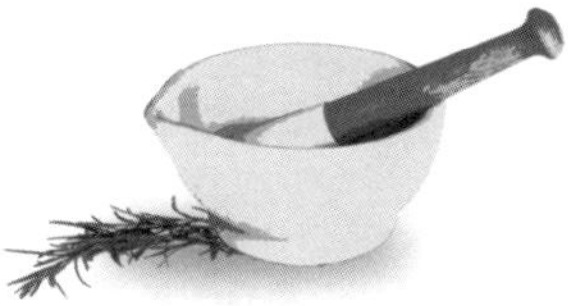

Blending Basics

You can blend essential oils for therapeutic reasons or just to make your own individual statement through a natural perfume. Decide what you want your scent to "say", then follow these basic guidelines, and combine with imagination, passion, and fun!

Below is a simple chart to help you get started.

	Essential Oil (common/botanical name)	Note (Top/Mid/ Base)	Number Drops
1			
2			
3			
4			
5			
What is the theme?			
What will you call this blend?			

Until you get a feel for blending, it may be easier to start with no more than 5 oils per blend, adding the essential oils—drop by drop. To know what oils will smell like when mixed together, use small tester strips of card stock and add the oils on the paper. It is imperative that you jot down exactly what oils and in what quantities you use.

Just like fine wine, essential oil blends improve with age. Let your blends age for a week or more and then retest for evolved scent. When happy with the aroma, store the blend in as small a bottle as possible; or you can immediately dilute it to make a perfume. The blended essential oils are diluted in a carrier oil, such as jojoba, almond, or sesame, using 15-30% essential oil to carrier oil (i.e., 15-10 drops essential oil to 70-85 drops carrier oil).

Perfumers use the terms top, middle, and base, to describe scents, based on their evaporation rate. They also use the following classifications to describe aroma:

- Anisic
- Balsamic
- Camphoraceous
- Chypre
- Citrus
- Fern
- Floral
- Forest-like
- Green
- Leather
- Oriental
- Powdery
- Resinous
- Spicy
- Woody

Although there are no hard and fast rules about oils and their notes, there are some basic guidelines. The complexity of some single essential oils allows them to fit into all of the note categories, depending on the other oils in the blend. Below is a chart describing the general characteristics of each note:

Note	Volatility/ Evaporation Rate	Description
Top	Most prominent up to 30 minutes to 1 or 2 hours after application.	"Head" notes. Fastest evaporation rate. Gives first impression of the blend. Aromatically sharp or pungent. Energetically uplifting, energizing, fresh; some are warming. Includes citrus, needle, eucalyptus, and mints.
Middle	Most prominent up to 2-4 hours after application.	"Heart" notes. Aromatically mellow and round. Gives body and balance to the blend. Often comprises 50% or more of the blend. Energetically fortifying, harmonizing, regulating, centering, soothing. Includes chamomile, lavender, geranium, and petitgrain.
Base	Most prominent up to 4-6 hours after application.	"Root" note. Slowest evaporation rate. Often acts as a fixative to hold the blend together. Aromatically deep, earthy, sensual. Gives depth to the blend. Energetically grounding, relaxing, supporting. Slower vibration inspires contemplation or mediation; encourages a deeper connection to our physical, sensual selves; and promotes sleep. Includes benzoin, balsams, myrrh, patchouli, and vetiver.

There are several techniques for blending, depending upon the blender:

- Combining essential oils for their effects (i.e., stimulating, euphoric, relaxing, etc.).

- Combining at least one top, one middle, and one base note as a basic blend, and adding additional scents as "bridging" notes and a fixative essential oil.

- Combining essential oils from the same plant part (i.e. flowers, citrus rinds, woods, etc.).

- Combining essential oils from the same botanical family.

- A combination of all of the above techniques.

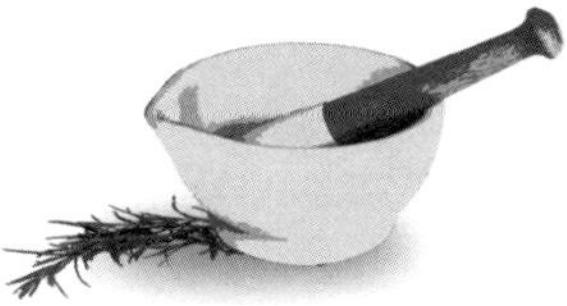

GLOSSARY OF TERMS

Amenorrhea	Absence of menstruation outside pregnancy in pre-menopausal women
Analgesic	Reduces or relieves pain
Anaphrodisiac	Eliminates or diminishes sexual desire
Antiallergenic	Not aggravating an allergy; tending to relieve or control allergic symptoms
Antibacterial	Prevents the growth of and kills bacteria
Anticoagulant	A substance that prevents the clotting of blood
Antidepressant	Reduces depression and helps uplift mood
Antifungal	Destroys fungal infections
Antihistamine	Counteracts histamine and allergic conditions
Antineuralgic	Helps soothe nerve pain
Anti-inflammatory	Reduces heat, redness, and swelling associated with inflammation
Antiparasitic	Destroys parasites

Antirheumatic	Helps ease arthritic symptoms such as musculoskeletal pain and inflammation
Antiseptic	Inhibits the growth of microorganisms
Antispasmodic	Relieves or prevents spasms or cramps
Antiviral	Weakens and kills viruses
Anxiolytic	A substance that relieves anxiety
Aphrodisiac	Enhances or stimulates erotic feelings
Astringent	Contracts, firms, and strengthens skin and other tissue and reduces secretions
Bronchodilator	Dilates the bronchial tube
Cardiotonic	Tones the heart muscle
Carminative	Promotes digestion and peristalsis, assists in expulsion of intestinal gas
Catarrh	Inflammation of mucous membranes, especially of the nose and throat
Cicatrizant	Promotes the healing of a wound and formation of scar tissue
Counterirritant	Agent that induces local inflammation to relieve inflammation in underlying or adjacent tissues
Decongestant	Relieves congestion

Dermatitis	Inflammation of the skin
Disinfectant	Kills infections and disease-producing micro organisms
Diuretic	A substance that tends to increase the discharge of urine
Dysmenorrhea	Difficult or painful menstruation
Dyspepsia	Difficult digestion
Edema	An excessive accumulation of serous fluid in tissue spaces or a body cavity
Emollient	Softens, soothes, and protects especially dry or chapped skin.
Emmenagogic	Promotes and regulates menstruation
Euphoric	Promotes a sense of well-being
Expectorant	Promotes elimination of excess mucous from the lungs and bronchial tubes
Fixative	A viscous (thick) oil with a very low evaporation rate, used in perfumery to stabilize and increase the "staying power" of a blend to hold the scent of a fragrance
Hepatic	Related to the liver

Hypotensive	Reduces blood pressure
Immunostimulant	An substance that stimulates an immune response
Insectifugal	Repels insects
Lactogenic	Promotes the secretion of milk
Mucolytic	Dissolves, digests, or liquifies mucus
Neat	To apply undiluted, and directly on skin
Neuralgia	Sharp, severe pain extending along a nerve or group of nerves
Neurotonic	An agent that improves the tone or force of the nervous system, or strengthens or stimulates an impaired nervous action
Nervine	Having an effect on the nervous system, such as calming and soothing
Oligomenorrhea	Abnormally light or infrequent menstruation

Parasympathetic Nervous System The part of the autonomic nervous system originating in the brain stem and the lower part of the spinal cord that, in general, inhibits or opposes the physiological effects of the sympathetic nervous system. Serves to slow the heart rate, increase the intestinal and gland activity, and relax the sphincter muscles.

Photosensitizing, phototoxic May cause a skin reaction such as burning, irritation, or pigment change upon exposure to ultraviolet light (sunlight, tanning lights)

Pruritis Itching

Regulating Helps balance and normalize body functions

Rheumatism Any of several pathological conditions of the muscles, tendons, joints, bones, or nerves, characterized by discomfort and disability

Rubefacient A substance that irritates the skin, causing redness

Sedative Relaxing, calming, soothing effects, promotes drowsiness

Sensitizing Capable of producing an irritation or allergic reaction

Spasmolytic Relieves convulsions, spasmodic pains, and cramps

Sympathetic nervous system The part of the autonomic nervous system originating in the thoracic and lumbar regions of the spinal cord that, in general, inhibits or opposes the physiological effects of the parasympathetic nervous system. Accelerates the heart rate, constricts blood vessels, and raises blood pressure.

Stimulant Invigorating, stimulating, energizing effects

Stomachic Strengthens, stimulates, and tones the stomach

Tonic Strengthens and invigorates the entire body or specific organs

Uterotonic An agent that overcomes relaxation of the muscular wall of the uterus; gives tone to the uterine muscle

Vulnerary Affects wound healing, skin regenerative

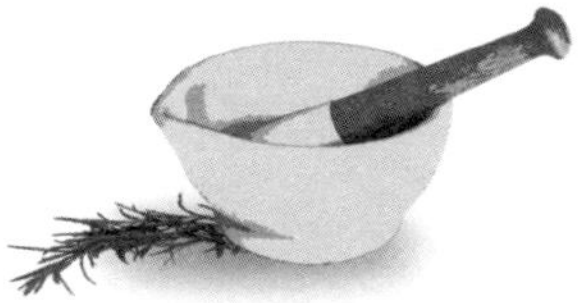

References and Suggested Reading List

Balacs, T., and Tisserand, R. *Essential Oil Safety: A Guide for Health Care Professionals*. London: Churchill Livingston, 1995.

Balz, Rodolphe. *The Healing Powers of Essential Oils*. Wisconsin: Lotus Light Productions, 1996.

Berwick, Ann. *Aromatherapy: A Holistic Guide*. Minnesota: Llewellyn Publications, 1996.

Blumenthal, Mark. *The ABC Clinical Guide to Herbs*. Texas: American Botanical Council, 2003.

Brinker, Francis. *Herb Contraindications and Drug Interactions*. Oregon: Eclectic Institute, Inc., 1997.

Buckle, Jane. *Clinical Aromatherapy in Nursing*. California: Singular Publishing Group, 1997.

Buckle, Jane. *Clinical Aromatherapy: Essential Oils in Practice*. London: Churchill Livingston, 2003.

Catty, Suzanne. *Hydrosols: The Next Aromatherapy*. Vermont: Healing Arts Press, 2001.

Cooksley, Valerie Gennari. *Aromatherapy: A Lifetime Guide to Healing with Essential Oils*. New Jersey: Prentice Hall, 1996.

Cunningham, Scott. *Magical Aromatherapy*. Minnesota: Llewellyn Publications, 1989.

Damian, Peter and Kate. *Aromatherapy Scent and Psyche*. Vermont: Healing Arts Press, 1997.

Dermaderosian, Ara. *Natural Products Handbook*. Missouri: Wolters Kluwer Health, Inc., 2001.

England, Allison. *Aromatherapy for Mother and Baby*. Vermont: Healing Arts Press, 1994.

Facts and Comparisons. *Guide to Popular Natural Products*. Missouri: Facts and Comparisons, 1999.

Foster, Steven. *Herbs for Your Health*. Colorado: Interweave Press, 1996.

Gattefosse, Rene-Maurice. *Gattefosse's Aromatherapy*. Essex: C. W. Daniel Co., 1993.

Green, Mindy. *Natural Perfumes*. Colorado: Interweave Press, 1999.

Hay, Louise. *You Can Heal Your Life*. California: Hay House, 1984.

Higley, Connie and Alan. *Reference Guide for Essential Oils*. Kansas: Abundant Health, 1998.

Hoffman, David. *The Herbal Handbook*. Vermont: Healing Arts Press, 1988.

Icon Health Publications, ed. *Aromatherapy: A Medical Dictionary, Bibliography, and Annotated Research Guide to Internet References*. California: Icon Health, 2003.

Keller, Erich. *Aromatherapy Handbook for Beauty, Hair, and Skin Care*. Vermont: Healing Arts Press, 1991.

Keville, Kathy, and Green, Mindy. *Aromatherapy: A Complete Guide to the Healing Art*. California: The Crossing Press, 1995.

Keville, Kathy. *Aromatherapy for Dummies*. California: IDG Books Worldwide, Inc., 1999.

Lavabre, Marcel. *Aromatherapy Workbook*. Vermont: Healing Arts Press, 1990.

Lawless, Julia. T*he Encyclopedia of Essential Oils*. Massachusetts: Element Books, Limited, 1992.

Lowe, David; Tisserand, Robert; and Clark, Sue. *Essential Chemistry for Safe Aromatherapy*. London: Churchill Livingston, 2002.

Mars, Brigitte. *Addiction-Free Naturally*. Vermont: Healing Arts Press, 2001.

McKenna, Dennis; Jones, Kenneth; and Hughes, Kerry. *Botanical Medicines: The Desk Reference for Major Herbal Supplements*. New York: Haworth Press Inc., 2002.

Mein, Carolyn. *Releasing Emotional Patterns with Essential Oils*. California: VisonWare Press, 1999.

Mojay, Gabriel. *Aromatherapy for Healing the Spirit*. New York: Henry Holt, 1996.

Monte, Tom. *World Medicine: The East West Guide to Healing Your Body*. New York: Putnam Publishing Group, 1993.

Olsen, Cynthia. *Birth of the Blue*. Colorado: Kali Press, 2000.

Olshevsky, Moshe, et al. *The Manual of Natural Therapy*. New York: Carol Publishing, 1993.

Pavia, Fabienne. *The World of Perfume*. New York: Knickerbocker Press, 1995.

Poth, Suzanne. *Tea Tree Oil for Health and Well-Being*. New York: Sterling Publishing Company, Inc., 1999.

Price, Shirley, and Price, Len. *Aromatherapy for Health Professionals*. New York: Churchill Livingstone, 1995.

Price, Shirley. *Aromatherapy for Common Ailments*. London: Gaia Books Ltd., 1991.

Price, Shirley. *Aromatherapy Workbook*. California: Thorsens, 1993.

Quality of Life Associates. *Aromatherapy Education Package*. Massachusetts: QLA, 1993.

Raiguel, Jill. Life Skill: *Keys to Effective Living*. Nevada: Marshall Educational Healing Solutions, Inc., 1999.

Rose, Jeanne, and Earle, Susan. *The World of Aromatherapy*. California: Frog, Ltd., 1996.

Rose, Jeanne. *Guide to 325 Essential Oils*. California: Jeanne Rose, 1994.

Schiller, Carol, and Schiller, David. *Aromatherapy Oils: A Complete Guide*. New York: Sterling Publishing Company, 1996.

Schnaubelt, Kurt. *Advanced Aromatherapy-The Science of Essential Oil Therapy*. Vermont: Healing Arts Press, 1998.

Schnaubelt, Kurt, et al. *Essential Oils and Cancer*. California: Terra Linda Scent and Image, 2000.

Schnaubelt, Kurt. *Medical Aromatherapy: Healing with Essential Oils*. California: Frog Ltd., 1999.

Schultz, Mona Lisa. *Awakening Intuition*. New York: Three Rivers Press, 1998.

Sellar, Wanda. *The Directory of Essential Oils*. Essex: C.W. Daniel Company, Ltd., 2001.

Stein, Diane. *The Natural Remedy Book for Women*. California: The Crossing Press, 1992.

Tisserand, Robert. *The Art of Aromatherapy*. Vermont: Healing Arts Press, 1977.

Tourles, Stephanie. *The Herbal Body Book*. Vermont: Storey Communications, Inc., 1994.

Tyler, Varro. *Herbs of Choice*. New York: Haworth Press, Inc., 1999.

Tyler, Varro. *The Honest Herbal*. New York: The Haworth Press, Inc., 1993.

Valnet, Jean. *The Practice of Aromatherapy*. Vermont: Healing Arts Press, 1990.

Vanderhaeghe, Lorna, and Karst, Karlene. *Healthy Fats for Life*. Kingston, Ontario: Quarry Health Books, 2003.

Watson, Franzesca. *Aromatherapy Blends and Remedies*. California: Thorsens, 1995.

Webb, Mark. *Bush Sense: Australian Essential Oils and Aromatic Compounds*. Adelaide, Australia: Griffin Press, 2000.

Wilson, Roberta. *A Complete Guide to Understanding and Using Aromatherapy for Vibrant Health and Beauty*. New York: Avery Publishing Group, 1995.

Worwood, Valerie Ann. *Aromatherapy for the Healthy Child: More Than 300 Natural, Non-Toxic, and Fragrant Essential Oil Blends*. California: New World Library, 2000.

Worwood, Valerie Ann. *The Complete Book of Essential Oils and Aromatherapy*. California: New World Library, 1991.

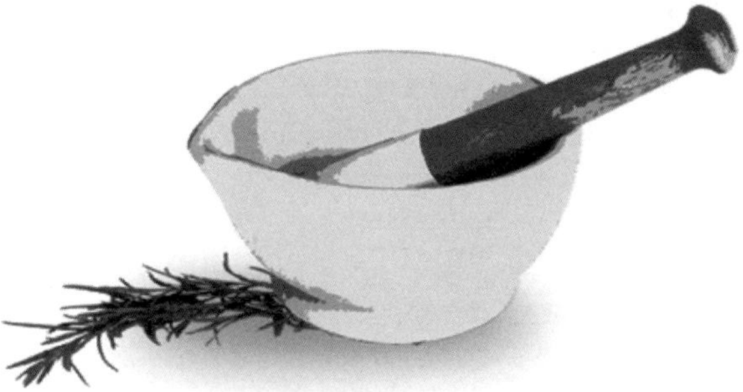

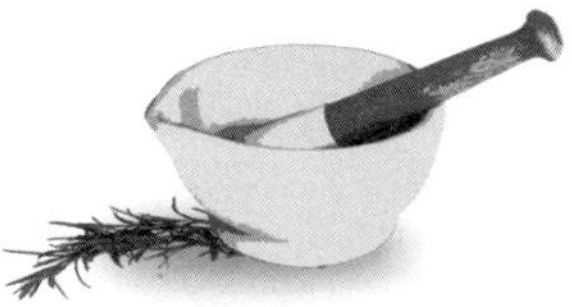

Informational Websites

http://dietary-supplements.info.nih.gov

Office of Dietary Supplements (ODS) supports research and disseminates research results in the area of dietary supplements. The ODS also provides advice to other federal agencies regarding research results related to dietary supplements.

http://www.altmedicine.com

Alternative Health News Online offers news pages that link some of the most informative and credible sites available on the Internet, with a substantial number of excellent conventional health sites, to provide a truly integrative approach.

http://www.askdrweil.com

DrWeil.com is a leading provider of online information and products for optimum health and wellness. Andrew Weil, MD, is a Harvard Medical School graduate who also holds an AB degree in biology (botany) from Harvard University. Dr. Weil is an internationally recognized expert on medicinal herbs, mind-body interactions and integrative medicine.

http://www.cancer.gov/cam

The **Office of Cancer Complementary and Alternative Medicine** (OCCAM) was established in October 1998 to coordinate and enhance the activities of the National Cancer Institute (NCI) in the arena of complementary and alternative medicine (CAM).

http://www.consumerlabs.com

ConsumerLab.com provides independent test results and information to help consumers and healthcare professionals evaluate health, wellness, and nutrition products.

http://www.datadiwan.de/index_e.htm

The **Datadiwan** is first and foremost a database where actual information on holistic medicine and frontier sciences can be accessed. Secondly, the Datadiwan is as a scientific discussion forum, where interested parties can discuss scientific topics with other like-minded people. And thirdly, the Datadiwan is a network which links research institutions and organizations worldwide.

http://www.fda.gov

The **U.S. Food and Drug Administration** is responsible for protecting the public health by assuring the safety, efficacy, and security of human and veterinary drugs, biological products, medical devices, our nation's food supply, cosmetics, and products that emit radiation. The FDA is also responsible for advancing the public health by helping to speed innovations that make medicines and foods more effective, safer, and more affordable and for helping the public get the accurate, science-based information needed to use medicines and foods to improve their health.

http://www.herbalgram.org

The **American Botanical Council** is an independent, nonprofit, international member-based organization providing education using science-based and traditional information to promote the responsible use of herbal medicine.

http://www.herbs.org

The **Herb Research Foundation** is a source of accurate, science-based information on the health benefits and safety of herbs, and expertise in sustainable botanical resource development.

http://www.holistickids.org/

HolisticKids.org is a site designed to provide information and resources for healthcare providers on complementary and alternative medicine use in children, exploring evidence, common problems, therapies, and practitioners.

http://www.holistic-online.com

Holisticonline.com is a comprehensive information website about health, featuring conventional, alternative, integrative, and mind-body medicine.

http://www.medherb.com

This site is generated by the **North American Institute of Medical Herbalism, Inc.**, and publishers of the Medical Herbalism. The purpose is to strengthen the herbal practitioner, to preserve and develop the science and art of herbal medicine, and to promote communication and sharing of clinical methods and experiences.

http://www.naturaldatabase.com

Natural Medicines Comprehensive Database has become the gold-standard, "go-to" source for reliable data in the natural medicine field.

http://www.nccam.nih.gov

The **National Center for Complementary and Alternative Medicine** (NCCAM) is dedicated to exploring complementary and alternative healing practices in the context of rigorous science, training complementary and alternative medicine (CAM) researchers, and disseminating authoritative information to the public and professionals.

http://www.pitt.edu/~cbw/altm.html

The **Alternative Medicine Homepage** is maintained by the Health Sciences Library System, University of Pittsburgh, to provide quality information in an objective manner, serve as a resource for locating quality CAM literature, and is a site to help individuals make informed decisions when selecting CAM modalities or therapies.

http://www.quackwatch.com/

Quackwatch, Inc., which was a member of Consumer Federation of America from 1973 through 2003, is a nonprofit corporation whose purpose is to combat health-related frauds, myths, fads, and fallacies. Its primary focus is on quackery-related information that is difficult or impossible to get elsewhere.

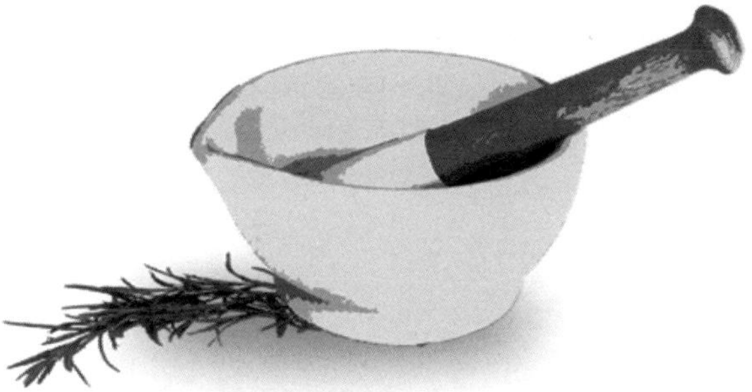

About Aroma Rx®, Inc.

We appreciate your interest in Aroma Rx®, Inc.! Our intention is to provide products of unsurpassed quality that enhance your health, vitality, and well-being. Aroma Rx®, Inc. distinguishes itself in the following ways:

Naturally Essential

Because our aromatherapy products are considered therapeutic, they are sourced, selected, manufactured, and marketed as if they were pharmaceutical products. Aroma Rx®, Inc. is committed to producing pure, consistent, reliable, efficacious quality products—100% natural oils that exactly duplicate the aromatic profile of the living plant source. Thus, we consider each point in depth:

- The Source
- The Selection
- Standardization
- Safety
- Substantiation
- Professional References

Our History

In 1998, Aroma Rx®, Inc. was founded to generate vitality through multiple uses of essential oils, with a commitment to global health transformation. At Aroma Rx®, Inc., we know that people are at their peak performance when they are well. The products and services of Aroma Rx®, Inc. are designed to support peak performance through wellness, relaxation, youthfulness, and serenity.

Aroma Rx®, Inc. provides essential oil products and health focused services through integrative medicine clinics, our Internet web site, and our distributors. All of our products are researched and developed by a registered pharmacist and a team of medically trained practitioners; this ensures quality, innovation, and safety. We are committed to professional, ethical, and accurate consumer education and affiliated quality products.

Aroma Rx®, Inc.'s Mission and Social Responsibility

Aroma Rx®, Inc.'s mission is to provide exceptional aromatherapy products and education that contribute to our customers' health and well-being. Aroma Rx®, Inc. operates in a socially responsible and environmentally sensitive manner by selecting the highest integrity and quality aromatherapy grade essential oils, never adulterated. Our sources are inspected, and our farmers maintain this same core value of respect for the universe. Aroma Rx®, Inc. respects the earth and promotes the spirit of people, their health, and community.

Aroma Rx®, Inc.'s Vision

Health transformation through education and products that empower individuals to be their own health advocates.

Aroma Rx®, Inc.'s Core Values

Integrity

- To select the highest integrity and quality aromatherapy grade essential oils, never adulterated.
- To provide meaningful work, fair compensation, and a safe, healthy work environment that encourages openness, creativity, self-discipline, and growth.
- To be distinctive in products and policies which honor and sustain our natural world.

Service

- To serve our customers by providing safe, effective, innovative, quality aromatherapy products.
- To build a relationship with our customers that extends beyond product usage and to develop enthusiastically satisfied customers.
- To create a new paradigm of holistic interconnectedness which facilitates mutual understanding and maximizes the synergistic benefits of a combined approach to health.

Excellence

- To respect, value, empower, and serve not only our customers, but also our co-workers, owners, suppliers, commissioned sales force, investors, and our community; to be concerned about and contribute to their well being and to operate with integrity, so as to be deserving of their trust.
- To acknowledge the value of each person's contribution to our goals, to foster teamwork in our tasks, and to treat each other with dignity and respect.
- To apply the highest standards of excellence to the selection, purchase, and manufacture of aromatherapy products.
- To work together to contribute to the long-term value and sustainability of our company.

For further information, contact

Aroma Rx® Inc/ The Aroma Shoppe
PO Box 331, 466 Bell Street
Los Alamos, CA 93440
Phone: 805-344-1314, Fax: 805-344-1334
www.aromarx.com

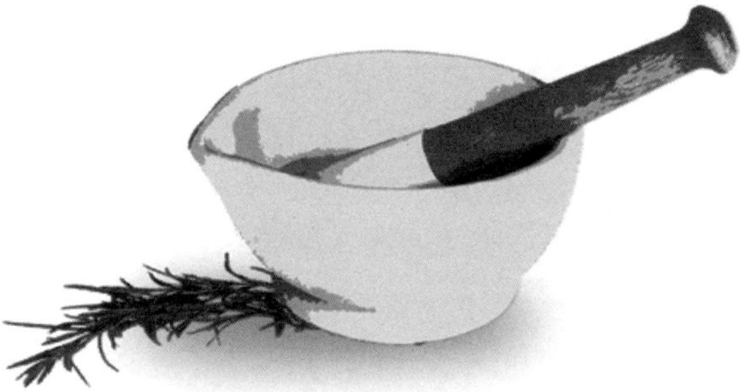

GIVE THE GIFT OF HEALTH!

Only the Essentials: A Concise Aromatherapy Reference Guide

☐ YES, I want ____ copies of *Only the Essentials: A Concise Aromatherapy Reference Guide* for $14.95 each.

☐ YES, I am interested in having Michele Williams offer a presentation to my company, association, school, or organization. Please send me information.

Include $3.95 shipping and handling for one book, plus $1.95 for each additional book. California residents must include applicable sales tax (7.75%). Payment must accompany orders. Allow two weeks for delivery.

My check or money order for $__________ is enclosed.

OR

Please charge my ☐ MasterCard ☐ Visa ☐ American Express

Card # ________________________ Expiration Date __________

Signature ______________________________________

Name ______________________________________

Organization ______________________________________

Mailing Address ______________________________________

City/State/Zip ______________________________________

Phone ______________________________________

E-mail ______________________________________

Fax ______________________________________

Call 805-344-1314

Make Checks payable to Aroma Rx®, Inc.
PO Box 331
Los Alamos, CA 93440
Fax: 805-344-1334

Visit us on the Web at www.aromarx.com

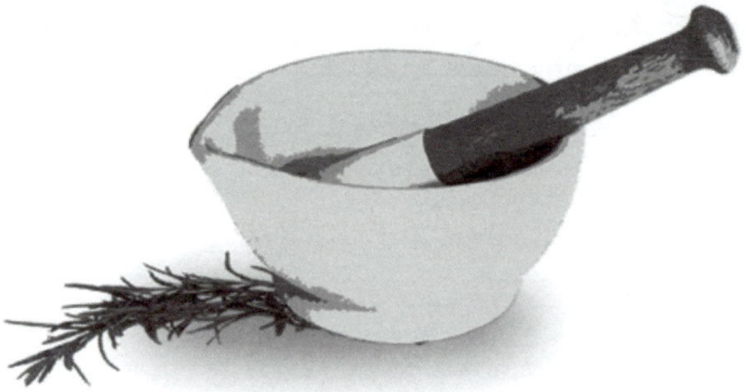